Welcome to ***"Diabetic Diet Cookbook for Seniors Over 50: 110+ Diabetes-Friendly Recipes for Vibrant Living After 50."*** *Whether you are newly diagnosed or have been managing diabetes for years, this cookbook is designed to help you navigate the journey of healthy eating with ease and enjoyment. As we age, our nutritional needs evolve, and it becomes increasingly important to make mindful choices that support our overall well-being.*

This book is more than just a collection of recipes; it is a guide to making delicious and nutritious meals that cater to the unique dietary needs of seniors managing diabetes. Each recipe is carefully crafted to balance flavors and nutrients, ensuring that you can enjoy your meals while maintaining stable blood sugar levels. From hearty breakfasts to satisfying dinners, and everything in between, these recipes are designed to be both flavorful and easy to prepare.

In addition to the recipes, you will find valuable tips on meal planning, grocery shopping, and understanding the nutritional requirements specific to seniors with diabetes. We have included practical advice on portion control, managing carb intake, and incorporating a variety of nutrient-dense foods into your daily diet. Our goal is to empower you with the knowledge and tools needed to take control of your health and live vibrantly.

As you explore the recipes in this cookbook, you will discover a variety of dishes that cater to different tastes and preferences. Whether you enjoy traditional comfort foods or are looking to try something new, there is something here for everyone. The recipes are simple enough for everyday cooking yet special enough to share with family and friends.

Living with diabetes does not mean giving up the joy of eating. With the right approach, you can continue to enjoy delicious meals that are good for your health. This cookbook is your companion on the path to vibrant living, offering over 110 diabetes-friendly recipes that will nourish your body and delight your taste buds.

*Thank you for choosing **"Diabetic Diet Cookbook for Seniors Over 50."** We hope this book inspires you to embrace a healthier lifestyle and discover the joy of eating well at any age. Let's embark on this journey together towards a healthier, happier you.*

Happy cooking!

Good advice diabetic diet for seniors over 50

1. Prioritize Whole Foods: Focus on fresh vegetables, fruits, whole grains, lean proteins, and healthy fats. These foods provide essential nutrients without causing large spikes in blood sugar levels.

2. Monitor Carbohydrate Intake: Carbohydrates have a significant impact on blood sugar. Choose complex carbs like whole grains and vegetables, and keep an eye on portion sizes to avoid blood sugar spikes.

3. Eat Regular, Balanced Meals: Consistent meal timing helps maintain stable blood sugar levels. Each meal should include a mix of carbohydrates, proteins, and healthy fats.

4. Stay Hydrated: Drink plenty of water throughout the day. Proper hydration is crucial for overall health and can help manage blood sugar levels.

5. Include Fiber-Rich Foods: Foods high in fiber, such as beans, whole grains, fruits, and vegetables, can help control blood sugar levels and promote digestive health.

6. Limit Processed and Sugary Foods: Avoid foods with added sugars and refined carbs. These can cause rapid increases in blood sugar levels. Opt for natural, unprocessed foods instead.

7. Watch Your Sodium Intake: High sodium intake can lead to high blood pressure, which is a concern for many seniors. Choose low-sodium options and flavor foods with herbs and spices.

8. Incorporate Healthy Fats: Include sources of healthy fats like avocados, nuts, seeds, and olive oil in your diet. These fats support heart health and provide sustained energy.

9. Stay Active: Regular physical activity helps manage blood sugar levels and overall health. Aim for at least 30 minutes of moderate exercise most days of the week, such as walking, swimming, or yoga.

10. Consult a Dietitian: A registered dietitian can provide personalized advice and help you create a meal plan that meets your individual health needs and preferences.

11. Monitor Blood Sugar Levels: Keep track of your blood sugar levels regularly to understand how different foods and activities affect them. This can help you make more informed dietary choices.

Breakfast
- *Menu:*
  - Scrambled eggs with spinach and tomatoes
  - Whole grain toast (or a low-carb alternative)
  - 1 small apple

- *Nutritional Focus:*
  - Proteins: Eggs provide essential protein without spiking blood sugar levels.
  - Carbohydrates: Whole grain toast or a low-carb option for fiber and sustained energy.
  - Fruits: Apple for natural sweetness and fiber.

Mid-Morning Snack
- *Menu:*
  - 10 almonds (or other nuts)
  - 1/2 cup Greek yogurt (unsweetened)

- *Nutritional Focus:*
  - Proteins and Healthy Fats: Nuts provide protein and healthy fats, while Greek yogurt offers probiotics and additional protein.

Lunch
- *Menu:*
  - Grilled chicken breast salad with mixed greens, cucumber, and bell peppers
  - Olive oil and vinegar dressing (or low-sugar dressing)
  - 1 small whole grain roll (optional)

- **Nutritional Focus:**
  - Lean Proteins: Chicken breast for protein without excessive fat.
  - Vegetables: Mixed greens, cucumber, and bell peppers for fiber and nutrients.
  - Healthy Fats: Olive oil in the dressing for heart health.

Afternoon Snack
- *Menu:*
  - 1 small piece of cheese (such as cheddar or mozzarella)
  - Carrot sticks or cucumber slices

- *Nutritional Focus:*
  - Proteins: Cheese for protein and calcium.
  - Vegetables: Carrot sticks or cucumber for fiber and vitamins.

Dinner
- Menu:
- Baked salmon with lemon and herbs
- Quinoa pilaf with mixed vegetables (like broccoli and bell peppers)
- Steamed asparagus

- Nutritional Focus:
- Omega-3 Fatty Acids: Salmon for heart health and inflammation reduction.
- Whole Grains: Quinoa for fiber and sustained energy.
- Vegetables: Mixed vegetables and asparagus for vitamins and minerals.

Evening Snack
- Menu:
- 1 small piece of dark chocolate (at least 70% cocoa)
- Herbal tea (unsweetened)

- Nutritional Focus:
- Antioxidants: Dark chocolate for antioxidants and heart health benefits.
- Hydration: Herbal tea for relaxation and hydration.

Additional Tips:
- Hydration: Throughout the day, drink plenty of water or herbal tea.
- Portion Control: Pay attention to portion sizes to avoid overeating.
- Physical Activity: Incorporate gentle exercise such as walking or yoga, based on individual capabilities.
- Medication Adherence: Take prescribed medications as directed by healthcare providers.

This plan provides a balanced approach to managing diabetes in seniors over 50, emphasizing nutrient-dense foods, portion control, and regular meals to support stable blood sugar levels and overall health. Adjust portions and specific foods based on individual dietary needs and preferences.

And there are more than 110 recipes from healthy breakfasts to nutritious lunches and light evenings for you.

With more than 100 recipes, you can freely create your own menu for a day

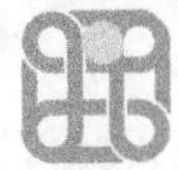

What is the total cooking time, including prep time?

Prep Time : ___________________

Cook Time : ___________________

Servings   : ___________________

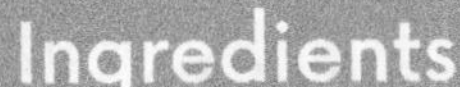

Ingredients:

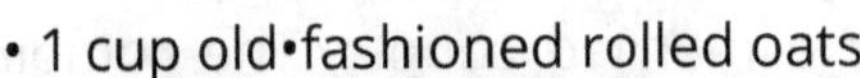

• 1 cup old•fashioned rolled oats
• 2 cups unsweetened almond milk (or low•fat milk)
• 1/4 tsp ground cinnamon
• 1 tbsp chopped walnuts or almonds
• 1 cup mixed fresh or frozen berries (such as blueberries, raspberries, blackberries)
• 1 tsp honey (optional)

Is the recipe easy to follow?

1. Oatmeal with Berries and Nuts

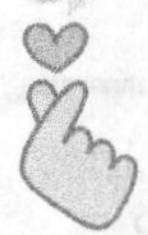

Procedure:

1. In a medium saucepan, combine the rolled oats and almond milk. Bring the mixture to a simmer over medium heat, stirring occasionally.

2. Reduce the heat to low and continue cooking the oatmeal for 5•7 minutes, or until it reaches your desired thickness, stirring frequently.

3. Remove the oatmeal from the heat and stir in the ground cinnamon.

4. Divide the oatmeal between two bowls. Top each serving with 1/2 cup of mixed berries, 1/2 tbsp of chopped nuts, and a drizzle of honey (if using).

This oatmeal dish is an excellent choice for seniors over 50 with diabetes. Oats are a complex carbohydrate that can help regulate blood sugar levels, while the berries and nuts provide fiber, healthy fats, and antioxidants.

The almond milk is a low•fat, low•carb dairy alternative that can help keep the carbohydrate content in check. The cinnamon also has potential benefits for blood sugar management.

Feel free to adjust the amounts of the ingredients to suit your individual dietary needs and preferences. You can also experiment with different types of berries and nuts to keep the dish varied and interesting.

Enjoy your Oatmeal with Berries and Nuts!

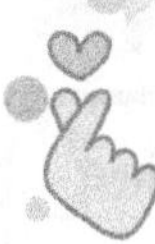

What are the critical points in the recipe (e.g., temperature control, timing)?

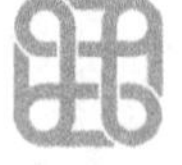

What is the total cooking time, including prep time?

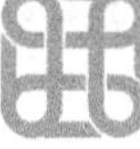

Prep Time : ___________________

Cook Time : ___________________

Servings : ___________________

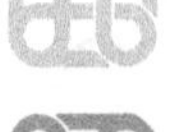

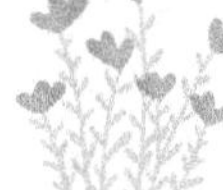

Ingredients:

- 2 cups plain Greek yogurt
- 2 tbsp chia seeds
- 1 cup mixed fresh berries (such as strawberries, blueberries, raspberries)
- 1 kiwi, peeled and sliced
- 1 tbsp honey (optional)

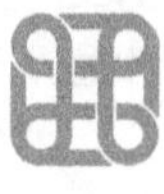
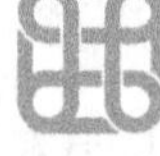
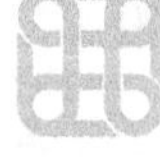
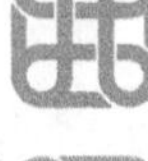
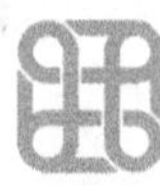

Is the recipe easy to follow?

2. Greek Yogurt with Chia Seeds and Fresh Fruit

1. In two serving bowls or glasses, divide the Greek yogurt evenly.

2. Sprinkle the chia seeds over the yogurt in each bowl.

3. Top the yogurt with the mixed fresh berries and sliced kiwi.

4. Drizzle the honey over the fruit and yogurt, if desired.

5. Serve immediately or refrigerate until ready to serve.

This healthy and delicious breakfast or snack is perfect for a married couple. The combination of creamy Greek yogurt, nutrient•dense chia seeds, and fresh, colorful fruit creates a satisfying and nutritious dish.

The chia seeds provide a boost of fiber, protein, and omega•3 fatty acids, while the fresh fruit adds natural sweetness and a variety of vitamins and antioxidants.

You can adjust the amounts of the ingredients to suit your preferences or the number of servings needed. Additionally, you can experiment with different types of fruit, such as mango, pineapple, or banana, to change up the flavors.

Enjoy your Greek Yogurt with Chia Seeds and Fresh Fruit!

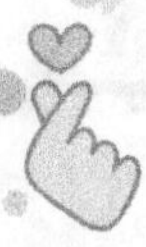

Procedure:

What are the critical points in the recipe (e.g., temperature control, timing)?

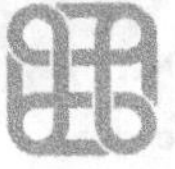

What is the total cooking time, including prep time?

Prep Time : ________________

Cook Time : ________________

Servings   : ________________

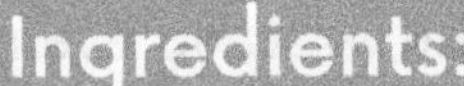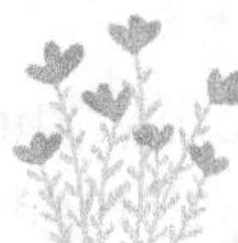

Ingredients:

• 4 large eggs
• 2 tbsp unsweetened almond milk (or low•fat milk)
• 1 tsp olive oil
• 1 cup sliced mushrooms
• 1 cup fresh spinach leaves
• 1/2 cup diced tomatoes
• 2 tbsp shredded low•fat cheddar cheese
• Salt and pepper to taste

Is the recipe easy to follow?

3. Vegetable Omelet with Spinach, Tomatoes, and Mushrooms

1. In a small bowl, whisk together the eggs and almond milk. Season with a pinch of salt and pepper.

2. Heat the olive oil in a nonstick skillet over medium heat.

3. Add the sliced mushrooms to the skillet and cook for 2•3 minutes, until they start to soften.

4. Add the fresh spinach leaves to the skillet and cook for 1•2 minutes, until the spinach is wilted.

5. Pour the egg mixture into the skillet, tilting the pan to allow the uncooked egg to flow to the edges.

6. When the bottom of the omelet is set, but the top is still slightly runny, sprinkle the diced tomatoes and shredded cheddar cheese over half of the omelet.

7. Use a spatula to fold the other half of the omelet over the filled half.

8. Cook for an additional 1•2 minutes, or until the omelet is set and the cheese is melted. Carefully slide the vegetable omelet onto a plate and serve immediately.

This omelet is a nutritious and satisfying meal for seniors over 50 with diabetes. The combination of protein•rich eggs, fiber•packed vegetables, and a small amount of low•fat cheese provides a balanced and blood sugar•friendly dish.

You can adjust the vegetable fillings based on your preferences or what you have on hand. Additionally, you can serve the omelet with a side of fresh fruit or a small green salad for a complete meal

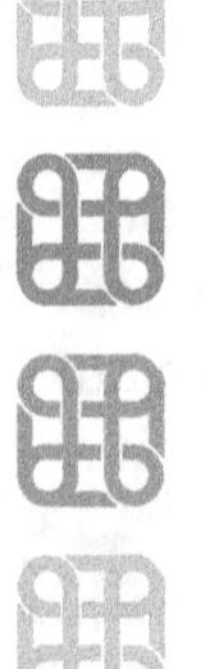

What is the total cooking time, including prep time?

Prep Time : _______________

Cook Time : _______________

Servings   : _______________

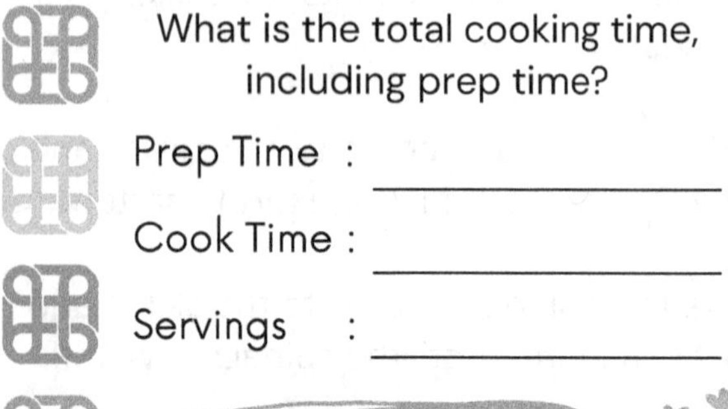

Ingredients:

- 2 slices whole grain bread
- 1/2 ripe avocado, mashed
- 1 large egg
- 1 tsp white vinegar
- Salt and pepper to taste

Is the recipe easy to follow?

4. Whole Grain Toast with Avocado and Poached Egg

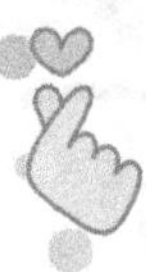

Procedure:

1. Bring a small saucepan of water to a gentle simmer over medium heat. Add the white vinegar to the water.

2. Crack the egg into a small bowl or cup. Gently slide the egg into the simmering water, being careful not to break the yolk. Poach the egg for 3•4 minutes, until the white is set but the yolk is still runny.

3. While the egg is poaching, toast the two slices of whole grain bread.

4. Spread the mashed avocado evenly over the toasted bread slices.

5. Using a slotted spoon, carefully remove the poached egg from the water and place it on top of the avocado toast.

6. Season the poached egg and avocado toast with salt and pepper to taste.

This meal provides a balance of complex carbohydrates, healthy fats, and protein, making it a nutritious choice. The whole grain toast provides fiber, the avocado offers heart•healthy monounsaturated fats, and the poached egg is a source of high•quality protein.

This recipe is suitable for a single serving, but you can easily scale it up to serve more people. Additionally, you can experiment with different types of whole grain bread or add other toppings, such as sliced tomatoes or a sprinkle of feta cheese, to customize the dish to your liking.

Enjoy your Whole Grain Toast with Avocado and Poached Egg!

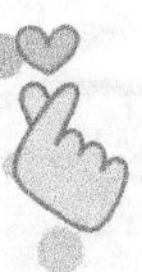

What are the critical points in the recipe (e.g., temperature control, timing)?

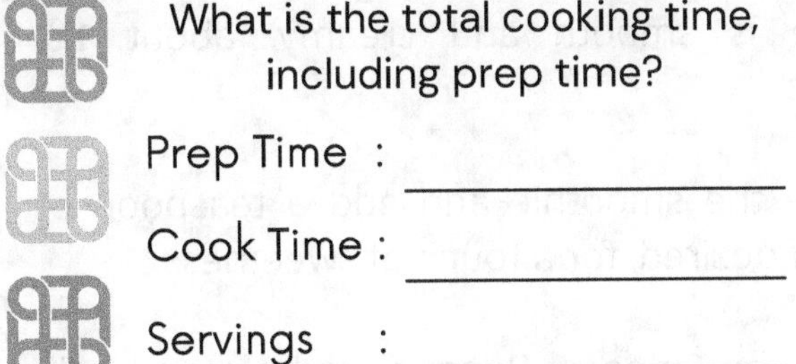

What is the total cooking time, including prep time?

Prep Time : _______________

Cook Time : _______________

Servings   : _______________

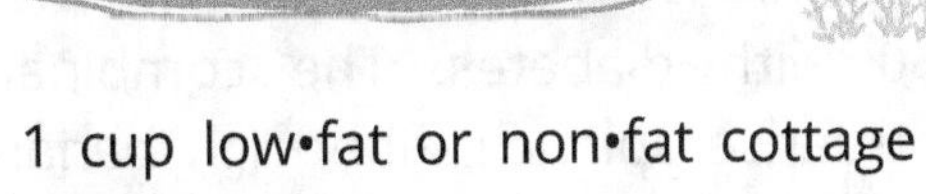

Ingredients:

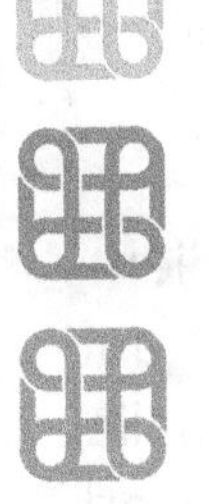

- 1 cup low•fat or non•fat cottage cheese
- 1 cup mixed fresh berries (such as blueberries, raspberries, and/or strawberries)
- 2 tbsp sliced or chopped almonds

Is the recipe easy to follow?

5. Cottage Cheese with Fresh Berries and Almonds

1. In a small bowl, place the cottage cheese.

2. Top the cottage cheese with the mixed fresh berries.

3. Sprinkle the sliced or chopped almonds over the top.

That's it! This simple, yet delicious, snack or light meal is ready to enjoy.

The combination of cottage cheese, fresh berries, and almonds provides a balance of protein, carbohydrates, and healthy fats. Cottage cheese is a great source of protein, while the berries offer fiber, vitamins, and antioxidants. The almonds add a crunchy texture and healthy monounsaturated fats.

This recipe is perfect for a quick and nutritious snack or light meal. It's versatile, so you can easily adjust the amounts of the ingredients to suit your preferences or appetite.

You can also experiment with different types of berries, such as blackberries or mixed berries, to change up the flavors. Additionally, you can try using other types of nuts, such as walnuts or pecans, in place of the almonds.

Enjoy your Cottage Cheese with Fresh Berries and Almonds!

What is the total cooking time, including prep time?

Prep Time : ________________

Cook Time : ________________

Servings : ________________

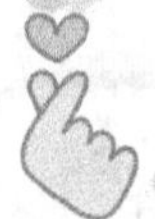

Ingredients:

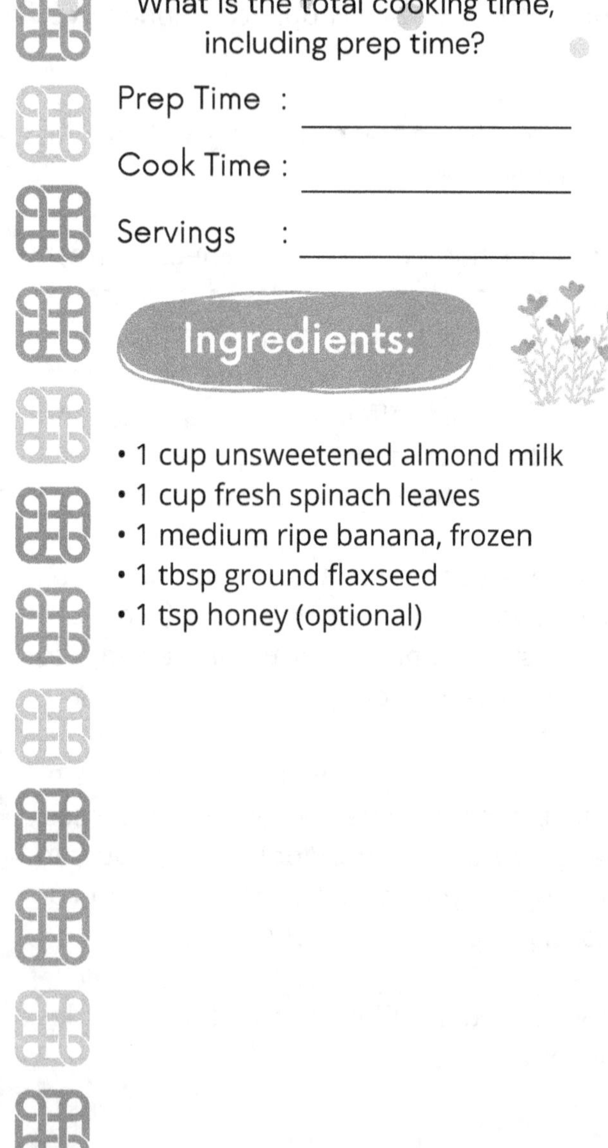

- 1 cup unsweetened almond milk
- 1 cup fresh spinach leaves
- 1 medium ripe banana, frozen
- 1 tbsp ground flaxseed
- 1 tsp honey (optional)

Is the recipe easy to follow?

6. Smoothie with Spinach, Banana, and Almond Milk

Procedure:

1. In a high•speed blender, combine the unsweetened almond milk, fresh spinach leaves, frozen banana, and ground flaxseed.

2. Blend the ingredients on high speed until the mixture is smooth and creamy, about 1•2 minutes.

3. Taste the smoothie and add a teaspoon of honey if desired, for a touch of sweetness.

4. Pour the Spinach, Banana, and Almond Milk Smoothie into a glass and enjoy immediately.

This smoothie is an excellent choice for seniors over 50 with diabetes. The combination of nutrient•dense spinach, fiber•rich banana, and protein•packed flaxseed provides a balanced and blood sugar•friendly meal or snack.

The unsweetened almond milk is a low•carb, low•fat dairy alternative that helps keep the carbohydrate content in check. The optional honey can be used sparingly to add a touch of sweetness, if desired.

You can adjust the amounts of the ingredients to suit your individual dietary needs and preferences. For example, you can use a smaller banana or add more spinach for a lower•carb option.

This smoothie is a great way to incorporate more vegetables, fruits, and healthy fats into your diet. Enjoy it as a quick and nutritious breakfast or snack.

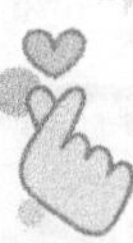

What are the critical points in the recipe (e.g., temperature control, timing)?

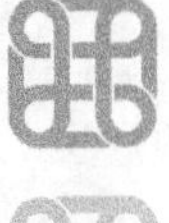

What is the total cooking time, including prep time?

Prep Time : _______________

Cook Time : _______________

Servings   : _______________

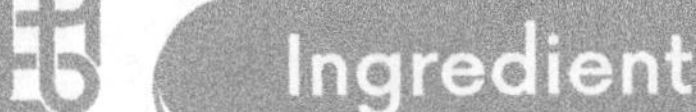
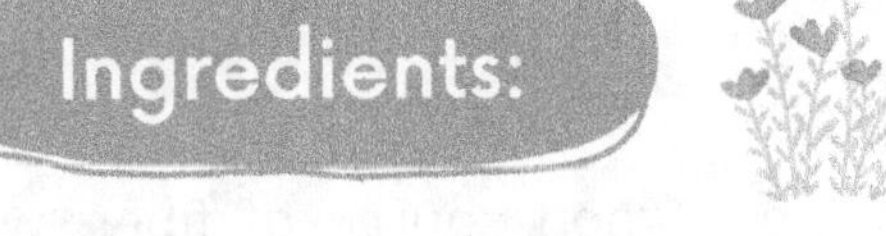

Ingredients:

• 2 medium carrots, peeled and cut into sticks

• 1 medium cucumber, cut into sticks

• 1/2 cup store•bought or homemade hummus

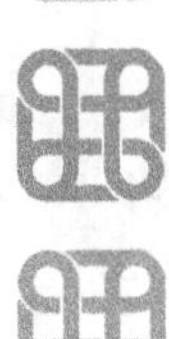
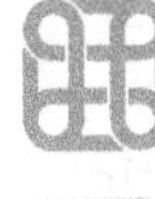
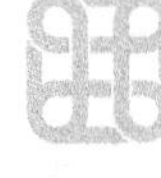
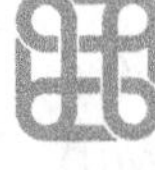
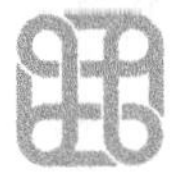

Is the recipe easy to follow?

7. Carrot and Cucumber Sticks with Hummus

1. Wash and peel the carrots. Cut them into long, thin sticks, about 4•5 inches long.

2. Wash the cucumber and cut it into long, thin sticks, about the same length as the carrot sticks.

3. Arrange the carrot and cucumber sticks on a plate or in a shallow bowl.

4. Serve the hummus in a small bowl or ramekin alongside the vegetable sticks.

This simple snack provides a balance of fiber, vitamins, and protein. The carrot and cucumber sticks offer a crunchy texture and a variety of nutrients, while the hummus provides a creamy, protein•rich dip.

Hummus is made from chickpeas, which are a good source of plant•based protein, fiber, and complex carbohydrates. It also contains healthy fats from ingredients like tahini (sesame seed paste) and olive oil.

This snack is a great option for a quick and healthy pick•me•up. It's also a versatile option that can be enjoyed as a light meal or as part of a larger spread of healthy snacks.

Feel free to experiment with different types of vegetables, such as bell peppers or celery, to dip in the hummus. You can also try making your own hummus at home for a more personalized flavor.

Enjoy your Carrot and Cucumber Sticks with Hummus!

What are the critical points in the recipe (e.g., temperature control, timing)?

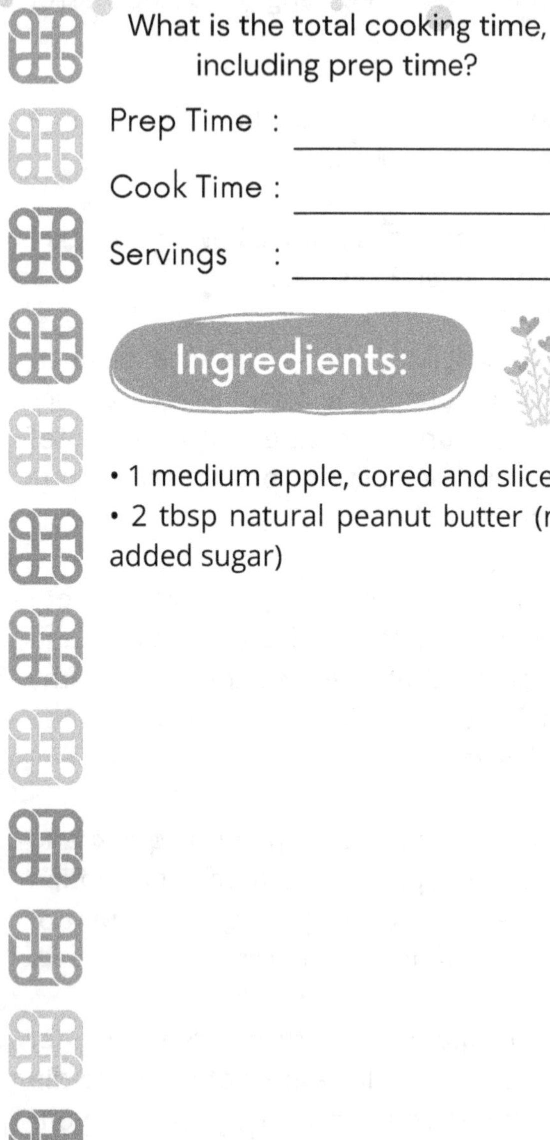

What is the total cooking time, including prep time?

Prep Time : _______________

Cook Time : _______________

Servings   : _______________

Ingredients:

- 1 medium apple, cored and sliced
- 2 tbsp natural peanut butter (no added sugar)

Is the recipe easy to follow?

8. Apple Slices with Peanut Butter

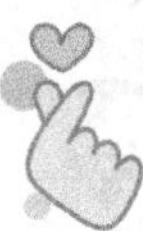

Procedure:

1. Wash the apple and slice it into thin wedges or rounds.

2. Arrange the apple slices on a plate or in a small bowl.

3. Serve the natural peanut butter in a small dish or dollop it directly onto the apple slices.

This simple snack is a great choice for seniors over 50 with diabetes. The combination of the apple's natural sweetness and the protein•rich peanut butter can help regulate blood sugar levels.

Apples are a good source of fiber, which can help slow the absorption of carbohydrates and prevent spikes in blood sugar. The peanut butter provides healthy fats and protein to help keep you feeling full and satisfied.

Be sure to choose a natural peanut butter without added sugars or other sweeteners, as these can contribute to a higher carbohydrate content.

You can adjust the portion sizes of the apple and peanut butter to suit your individual dietary needs and preferences. Some seniors may prefer to use a smaller apple or a reduced•fat peanut butter.

This snack is easy to prepare and can be enjoyed as a quick pick•me•up or as part of a balanced meal. Enjoy your Apple Slices with Peanut Butter!

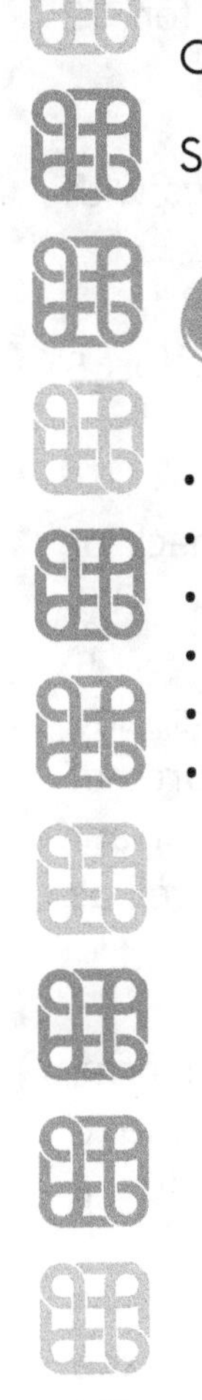

What are the critical points in the recipe (e.g., temperature control, timing)?

What is the total cooking time, including prep time?

Prep Time : _______________

Cook Time : _______________

Servings   : _______________

Ingredients:

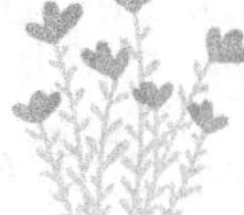

• 1/4 cup raw almonds
• 1/4 cup raw walnuts
• 2 tbsp raw pumpkin seeds
• 2 tbsp raw sunflower seeds
• 1 tbsp chia seeds
• 1 tbsp ground flaxseed

Is the recipe easy to follow?

9. Mixed Nuts and Seeds

Procedure:

1. In a small bowl, combine the raw almonds, walnuts, pumpkin seeds, sunflower seeds, chia seeds, and ground flaxseed.

2. Stir the mixture to evenly distribute the nuts and seeds.

That's it! Your Mixed Nuts and Seeds snack is ready to enjoy.

This combination of nuts and seeds provides a nutrient•dense and satisfying snack for seniors over 50 with diabetes. Here's why it's a great choice:

• Nuts and seeds are high in healthy fats, protein, fiber, and various vitamins and minerals. They can help regulate blood sugar levels and provide long•lasting energy.

• Almonds and walnuts are rich in monounsaturated and polyunsaturated fats, which can help improve heart health.

• Pumpkin seeds and sunflower seeds are good sources of magnesium, a mineral that plays a role in blood sugar control.

• Chia seeds and ground flaxseed provide additional fiber and omega•3 fatty acids, which have anti•inflammatory properties.

You can adjust the ratios of the nuts and seeds based on your personal preferences. Additionally, you can add a small amount of unsweetened coconut flakes or a sprinkle of cinnamon for extra flavor.

Portion control is important, so stick to the recommended serving size of 1/4 cup. Enjoy your Mixed Nuts and Seeds as a healthy snack or add it to your diabetic•friendly meals.

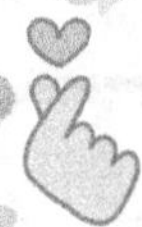

What are the critical points in the recipe (e.g., temperature control, timing)?

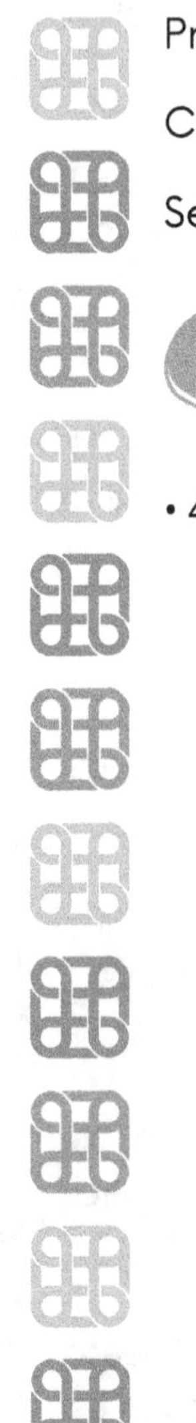

What is the total cooking time, including prep time?

Prep Time : _______________

Cook Time : _______________

Servings : _______________

Ingredients:

• 4 large eggs

Is the recipe easy to follow?

10. Hard·Boiled Eggs

1. Place the eggs in a single layer in a saucepan and cover with cold water by 1 inch.

2. Bring the water to a boil over high heat.

3. Once the water reaches a rolling boil, remove the pan from the heat and cover with a lid.

4. Let the eggs sit in the hot water for 12 minutes for hard·boiled eggs.

5. Drain the hot water and cover the eggs with cold water to stop the cooking process.

6. Let the eggs sit in the cold water for 5 minutes.

7. Peel the eggs and enjoy them as a snack or use them in other recipes.

Hard·boiled eggs are a simple, nutritious, and versatile snack. They are an excellent source of protein, and the yolks also contain important nutrients like vitamins A, D, and B12, as well as choline.

This recipe yields hard·boiled eggs with firm, cooked yolks. You can adjust the cooking time to your preference, such as 10 minutes for a softer, more jammy yolk.

Hard·boiled eggs can be stored in the refrigerator for up to 1 week, making them a convenient and easy·to·prepare snack. They can be enjoyed on their own, added to salads, or used in recipes like deviled eggs.

Remember to always use fresh, high·quality eggs for the best results. Enjoy your hard·boiled eggs!

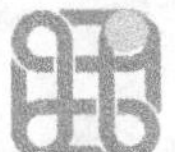 What are the critical points in the recipe (e.g., temperature control, timing)?

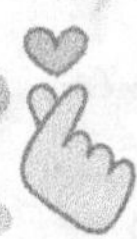

What is the total cooking time, including prep time?

Prep Time : ________________

Cook Time : ________________

Servings   : ________________

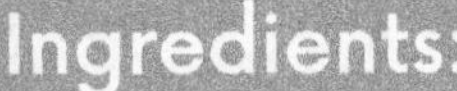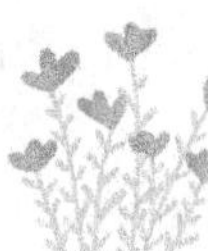
Ingredients:

• 1 cup plain Greek yogurt (full•fat or low•fat)
• 1 tablespoon ground flax seeds
• 1 teaspoon honey (optional)
• Fresh berries (such as blueberries, raspberries, or strawberries) • about 1/2 cup

1. In a bowl, combine the Greek yogurt and ground flax seeds. Stir well to mix.

2. If desired, drizzle the honey over the yogurt mixture and stir to incorporate.

3. Top the yogurt with the fresh berries.

Nutritional Benefits:
• Greek yogurt is high in protein, which is important for seniors to maintain muscle mass.

• Flax seeds are a good source of fiber, omega•3 fatty acids, and antioxidants, which can help manage blood sugar levels.

• Berries are low in carbs and high in fiber, vitamins, and antioxidants, making them a great choice for a diabetic•friendly snack.

• The honey (if used) provides a touch of sweetness without spiking blood sugar too much.

This simple, nutrient•dense snack can be a great option for seniors with diabetes, as it provides a balance of protein, fiber, and healthy fats to help regulate blood sugar levels.

Is the recipe easy to follow?

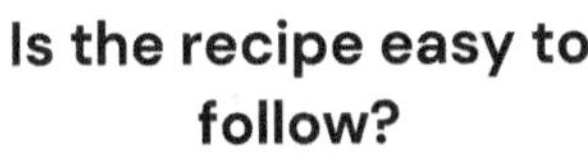
11. Greek Yogurt with Flax Seeds

What is the total cooking time, including prep time?

Prep Time : ______________

Cook Time : ______________

Servings   : ______________

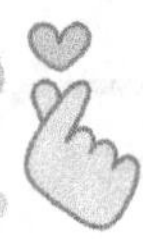

Ingredients:

• 4•6 celery stalks, washed and cut into 4•inch sticks
• 1 cup low•fat or non•fat cottage cheese

Is the recipe easy to follow?

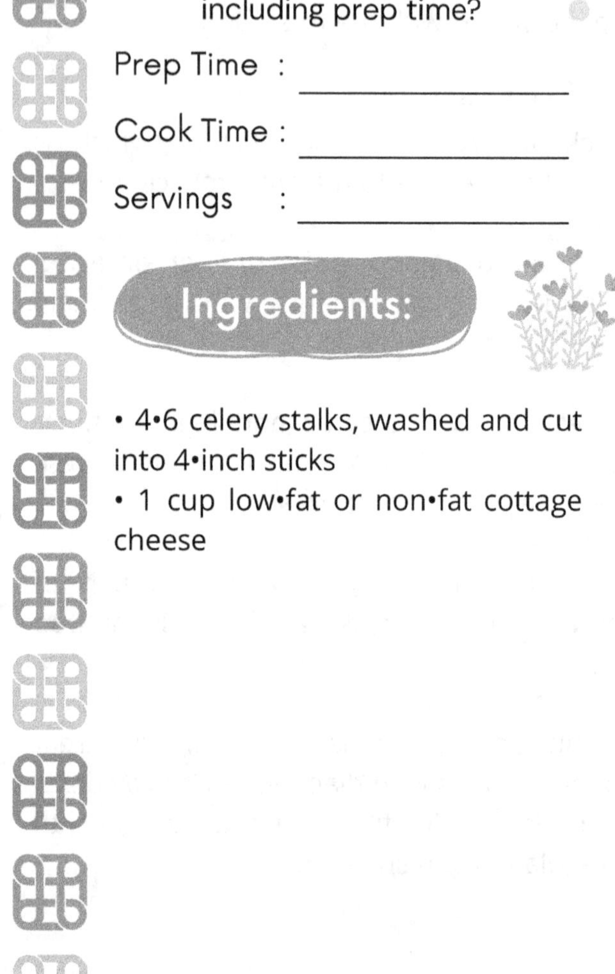

12. Celery Sticks with Cottage Cheese

Procedure:

1. Wash the celery stalks and cut them into 4•inch sticks.

2. Scoop a small amount of cottage cheese (about 2•3 tablespoons) onto each celery stick.

3. Serve immediately or refrigerate until ready to eat.

Tips:
• For extra flavor, you can sprinkle the cottage cheese with a bit of dried herbs, such as dill, chives, or parsley.

• You can also use flavored cottage cheese, such as garlic & herb or pineapple.

• This makes a great healthy snack or light appetizer. The combination of the crunchy celery and creamy cottage cheese is delicious.

!

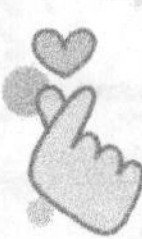

Procedure:

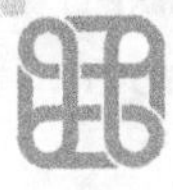
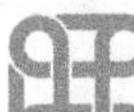

What is the total cooking time,
including prep time?

Prep Time : _______________

Cook Time : _______________

Servings   : _______________

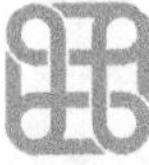

Ingredients:

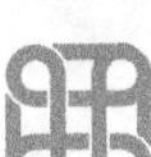
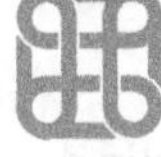
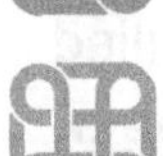
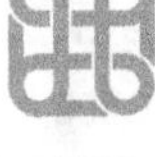

• 1 cup cooked quinoa, cooled
• 1 (15 oz) can chickpeas, rinsed and drained
• 1 cup diced cucumber
• 1 cup cherry or grape tomatoes, halved
• 1/4 cup chopped fresh parsley
• 2 tbsp olive oil
• 2 tbsp lemon juice
• 1 tsp Dijon mustard
• 1/4 tsp salt
• 1/4 tsp black pepper

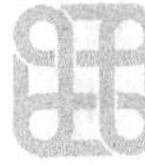
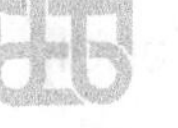
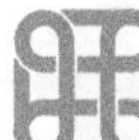
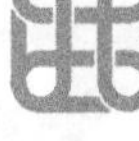
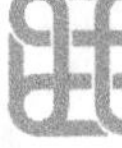
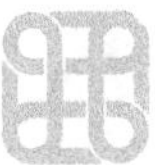
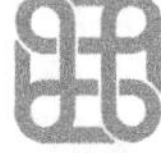
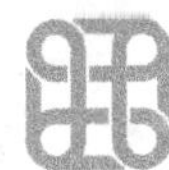

Is the recipe easy to follow?

13. *Quinoa Salad with Chickpeas, Cucumber, and Tomatoes*

1. In a large bowl, combine the cooked quinoa, chickpeas, cucumber, tomatoes, and parsley.

2. In a small bowl, whisk together the olive oil, lemon juice, Dijon mustard, salt, and pepper.

3. Pour the dressing over the quinoa salad and toss gently to coat.

4. Refrigerate for at least 30 minutes to allow the flavors to blend.

Nutrition Info (per serving):
Calories: 200
Carbs: 25g
Fiber: 5g
Protein: 7g
Fat: 8g
Sodium: 270mg

This quinoa salad is high in fiber, protein, and healthy fats, making it a great diabetic•friendly option. The vegetables provide vitamins, minerals, and antioxidants. Feel free to adjust the amounts of ingredients to your taste preferences.

Procedure:

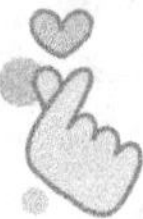

1. Make the balsamic vinaigrette by whisking together all the dressing ingredients in a small bowl. Set aside.

2. In a large salad bowl, arrange the mixed greens, grilled chicken, tomatoes, cucumber, and feta cheese.

3. Drizzle the balsamic vinaigrette over the salad and toss gently to coat.

Nutrition Info (per serving):
Calories: 250
Carbs: 12g
Fiber: 4g
Protein: 26g
Fat: 12g
Sodium: 450mg

This salad is high in protein from the grilled chicken, and the mixed greens provide fiber, vitamins, and minerals. The balsamic vinaigrette is a light, flavorful dressing that is low in calories and carbs. This makes a great diabetic•friendly main dish salad.

You can adjust the portion sizes or add/substitute ingredients to your liking. !

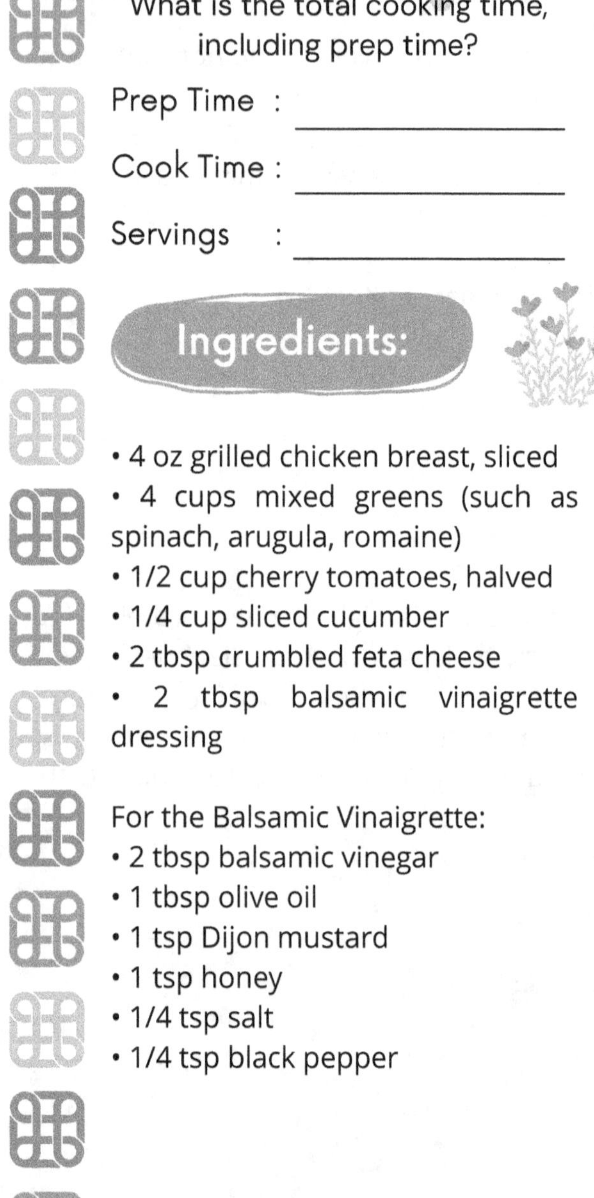

What is the total cooking time, including prep time?

Prep Time : _________________

Cook Time : _________________

Servings   : _________________

Ingredients:

• 4 oz grilled chicken breast, sliced
• 4 cups mixed greens (such as spinach, arugula, romaine)
• 1/2 cup cherry tomatoes, halved
• 1/4 cup sliced cucumber
• 2 tbsp crumbled feta cheese
• 2 tbsp balsamic vinaigrette dressing

For the Balsamic Vinaigrette:
• 2 tbsp balsamic vinegar
• 1 tbsp olive oil
• 1 tsp Dijon mustard
• 1 tsp honey
• 1/4 tsp salt
• 1/4 tsp black pepper

Is the recipe easy to follow?

14. Grilled Chicken Salad with Mixed Greens and Balsamic Vinaigrette

What are the critical points in the recipe (e.g., temperature control, timing)?

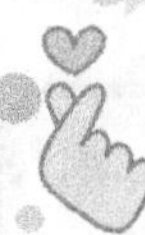

What is the total cooking time, including prep time?

Prep Time : _______________

Cook Time : _______________

Servings   : _______________

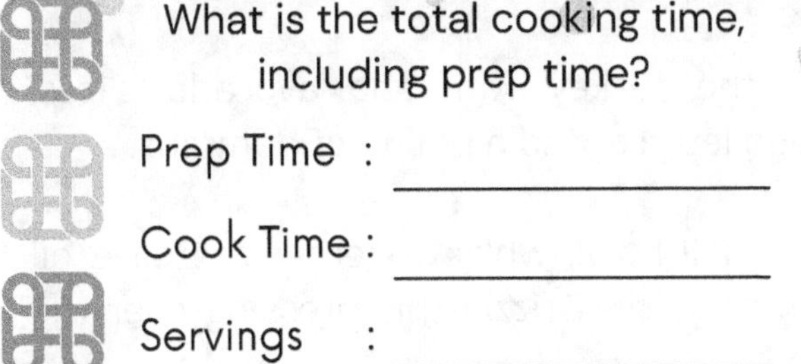

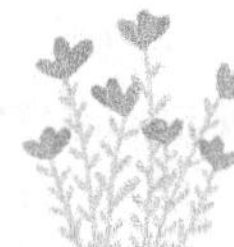

- 1 cup dry brown or green lentils, rinsed
- 4 cups low•sodium vegetable or chicken broth
- 1 tbsp olive oil
- 1 onion, diced
- 2 carrots, peeled and diced
- 2 celery stalks, diced
- 3 garlic cloves, minced
- 1 tsp ground cumin
- 1 tsp dried oregano
- 1/4 tsp red pepper flakes (optional)
- Salt and pepper to taste
- 2 cups chopped kale or spinach
- 1 (15 oz) can diced tomatoes

Is the recipe easy to follow?

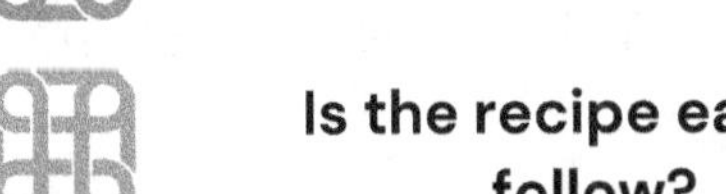

15. Lentil Soup with Vegetables

1. In a large pot, bring the lentils and broth to a boil over high heat. Reduce heat to medium•low, cover and simmer for 15•20 minutes until lentils are tender.

2. In a separate skillet, heat the olive oil over medium heat. Add the onion, carrots, celery and garlic. Sauté for 5•7 minutes until vegetables are softened.

3. Add the sautéed vegetables, cumin, oregano, red pepper flakes (if using), salt and pepper to the pot with the cooked lentils. Stir to combine.

4. Stir in the chopped kale/spinach and diced tomatoes. Simmer for an additional 5•10 minutes until greens are wilted and flavors have melded.

5. Taste and adjust seasonings as needed. Serve hot.

Nutrition Info (per serving):
Calories: 250
Carbs: 35g
Fiber: 12g
Protein: 15g
Fat: 6g
Sodium: 350mg

This lentil soup is packed with fiber, protein, and nutrients from the vegetables. It's a great diabetic•friendly meal that is easy to make. You can adjust the spices or add other veggies to your liking.

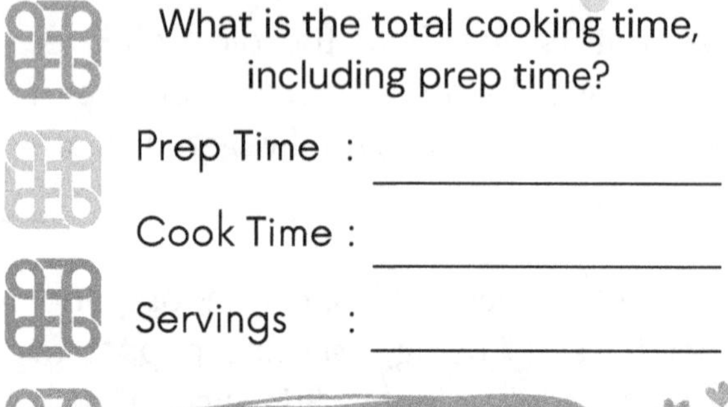

What is the total cooking time, including prep time?

Prep Time : _______________

Cook Time : _______________

Servings   : _______________

Ingredients:

- 1 (8·inch) whole wheat tortilla
- 2·3 oz sliced turkey breast
- 1/2 avocado, sliced
- 1/4 cup shredded lettuce
- 1 tbsp hummus
- 1 tsp olive oil
- 1 tsp lemon juice
- Salt and pepper to taste

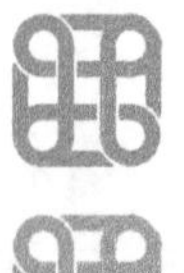
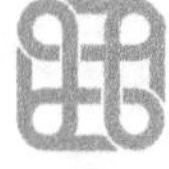
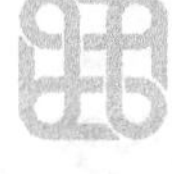
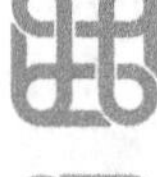
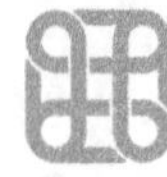

Is the recipe easy to follow?

☺   ☹

16. Turkey and Avocado Wrap in Whole Wheat Tortilla

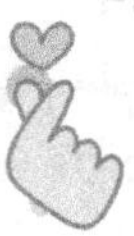

Procedure:

1. Lay the whole wheat tortilla flat on a clean surface.

2. Layer the turkey slices down the center of the tortilla.

3. Top the turkey with the avocado slices, shredded lettuce, and a dollop of hummus.

4. In a small bowl, whisk together the olive oil and lemon juice. Drizzle this dressing over the filling.

5. Season with a pinch of salt and pepper.

6. Fold the bottom of the tortilla up over the filling, then fold in the sides and continue rolling up tightly into a wrap.

7. Cut the wrap in half diagonally and serve.

Nutrition Info (per serving):
Calories: 300
Carbs: 25g
Fiber: 7g
Protein: 20g
Fat: 15g
Sodium: 550mg

This turkey and avocado wrap is a great diabetic·friendly option. The whole wheat tortilla provides complex carbs and fiber, while the turkey and avocado offer protein and healthy fats. The hummus adds creaminess without too many carbs. This makes a satisfying and nutritious lunch or snack.

You can adjust the portion sizes or swap in different veggies to your liking. !

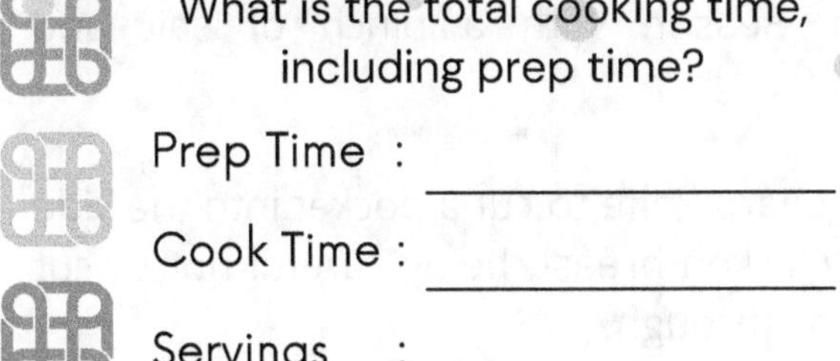

What is the total cooking time, including prep time?

Prep Time : ___________________

Cook Time : ___________________

Servings   : ___________________

Ingredients:

- 4 medium bell peppers (any color)
- 1 lb lean ground beef (93% lean or higher)
- 1 cup cooked brown rice
- 1 small onion, diced
- 2 cloves garlic, minced
- 1 (14.5 oz) can diced tomatoes
- 1 tsp dried oregano
- 1/2 tsp ground cumin
- 1/4 tsp red pepper flakes (optional)
- Salt and pepper to taste
- 1/2 cup shredded low·fat cheddar cheese

Is the recipe easy to follow?

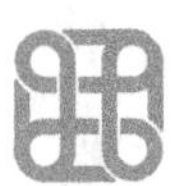

17. Stuffed Bell Peppers with Brown Rice and Lean Ground Beef

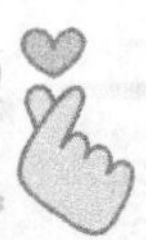

Procedure:

1. Preheat oven to 375°F. Cut the tops off the bell peppers and remove the seeds and membranes. Place the peppers in a baking dish.

2. In a skillet over medium heat, cook the ground beef, onion, and garlic until beef is browned and onions are translucent, about 5·7 minutes. Drain any excess fat.

3. Stir in the cooked brown rice, diced tomatoes, oregano, cumin, red pepper flakes (if using), and season with salt and pepper.

4. Spoon the beef and rice mixture evenly into the hollowed·out bell peppers. Top each pepper with a sprinkle of shredded cheddar cheese.

5. Cover the baking dish with foil and bake for 30·35 minutes, until the peppers are tender.

6. Remove the foil and bake for an additional 5 minutes to melt the cheese.

7. Serve the stuffed peppers warm.

Nutrition Info (per serving):
Calories: 300
Carbs: 25g
Fiber: 6g
Protein: 28g
Fat: 12g
Sodium: 450mg

This stuffed pepper dish is high in protein, fiber, and nutrients, making it a great diabetic·friendly meal. The lean ground beef, brown rice, and vegetables provide a balanced and satisfying dinner. Adjust the spices to your taste preferences.

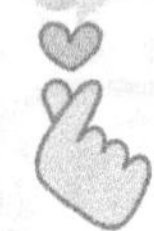

What are the critical points in the recipe (e.g., temperature control, timing)?

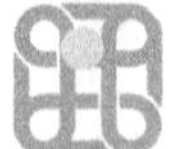

What is the total cooking time, including prep time?

Prep Time : ___________________

Cook Time : ___________________

Servings   : ___________________

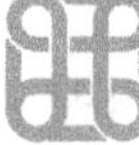

Ingredients:

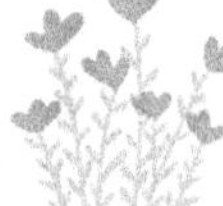

- 4 boneless, skinless chicken breasts
- 1 cup fresh spinach, chopped
- 1/2 cup crumbled feta cheese
- 2 tbsp cream cheese, softened
- 1 garlic clove, minced
- 1/4 tsp dried oregano
- Salt and pepper to taste
- 1 tbsp olive oil

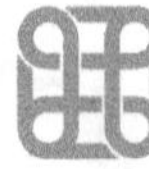
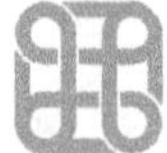
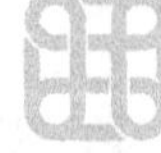
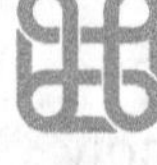
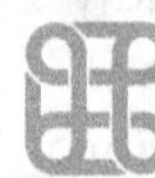

Is the recipe easy to follow?

18. Spinach and Feta Stuffed Chicken Breast

1. Preheat oven to 400°F. Lightly grease a baking dish or line with parchment paper.

2. In a small bowl, mix together the chopped spinach, feta cheese, cream cheese, garlic, and oregano. Season with a pinch of salt and pepper.

3. Use a sharp knife to cut a pocket into the side of each chicken breast, being careful not to cut all the way through.

4. Stuff each chicken breast with about 2•3 tablespoons of the spinach and feta mixture, pressing it into the pocket.

5. Heat the olive oil in a large skillet over medium•high heat. Sear the stuffed chicken breasts for 2•3 minutes per side to get a nice golden brown crust.

6. Transfer the seared chicken breasts to the prepared baking dish.

7. Bake for 20•25 minutes, until the chicken is cooked through and the internal temperature reaches 165°F.

8. Let the chicken rest for 5 minutes before serving.

This spinach and feta stuffed chicken breast is a delicious and healthy main dish. The creamy spinach and feta filling complements the lean chicken perfectly. Serve it with a side of roasted vegetables or a fresh salad for a complete diabetic•friendly meal.

!

What are the critical points in the recipe (e.g., temperature control, timing)?

What is the total cooking time, including prep time?

Prep Time : ________________

Cook Time : ________________

Servings   : ________________

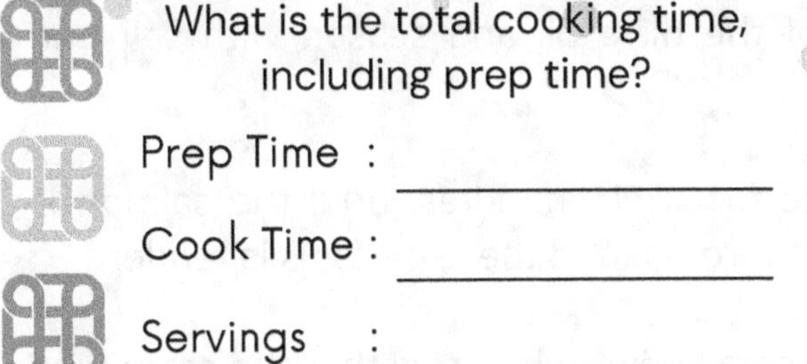

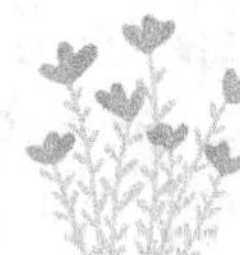

• 1 head of cauliflower, riced (about 4 cups riced cauliflower)
• 1 block (14 oz) extra•firm tofu, cubed
• 2 tbsp sesame oil
• 1 onion, diced
• 2 cloves garlic, minced
• 1 cup sliced mushrooms
• 1 cup chopped broccoli florets
• 2 tbsp low•sodium soy sauce or tamari
• 1 tsp rice vinegar
• 1 tsp grated fresh ginger
• 1/4 tsp red pepper flakes (optional)
• Salt and pepper to taste
• 2 tbsp chopped green onions (for garnish)

Is the recipe easy to follow?

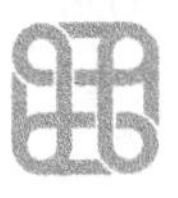  

19. Cauliflower Rice Stir•Fry with Tofu

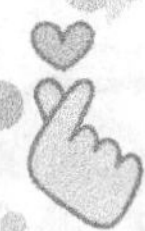

1. If using a whole head of cauliflower, pulse it in a food processor until it resembles rice•sized pieces. Measure out 4 cups of riced cauliflower.

2. In a large skillet or wok, heat the sesame oil over medium•high heat. Add the cubed tofu and cook for 3•4 minutes per side until lightly browned. Remove tofu from the pan and set aside.

3. In the same pan, sauté the onion and garlic for 2•3 minutes until fragrant.

4. Add the riced cauliflower, mushrooms, and broccoli. Stir•fry for 5•7 minutes until the vegetables are tender•crisp.

5. Return the cooked tofu to the pan. Add the soy sauce, rice vinegar, ginger, and red pepper flakes (if using). Toss everything together and cook for 2•3 more minutes.

6. Season with salt and pepper to taste.

7. Serve the cauliflower rice stir•fry hot, garnished with chopped green onions.

Nutrition Info (per serving):
Calories: 220
Carbs: 15g
Fiber: 5g
Protein: 16g
Fat: 13g
Sodium: 350mg

This cauliflower rice stir•fry is a great diabetic•friendly meal. The riced cauliflower provides a low•carb base, while the tofu, vegetables, and Asian•inspired seasonings make it flavorful and satisfying. Adjust the vegetable amounts to your liking.

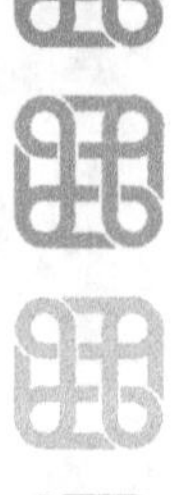

What is the total cooking time, including prep time?

Prep Time : _______________

Cook Time : _______________

Servings : _______________

Ingredients:

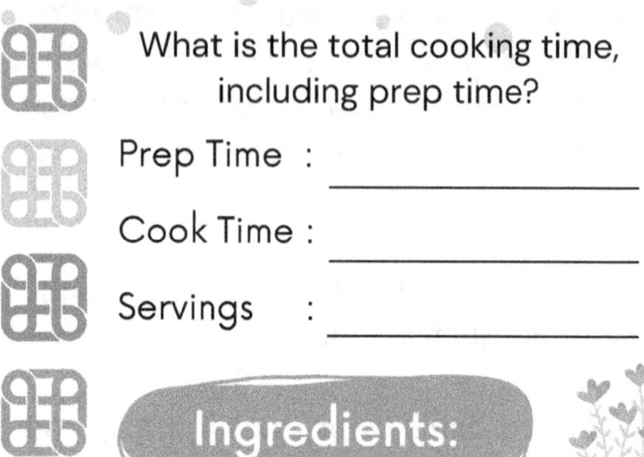

- 4 (4 oz) salmon fillets
- 1 lb asparagus, trimmed
- 1 cup cooked quinoa
- 2 tbsp olive oil, divided
- 1 tbsp lemon juice
- 1 tsp Dijon mustard
- 1 garlic clove, minced
- 1/4 tsp dried dill
- Salt and pepper to taste

Is the recipe easy to follow?

20. Baked Salmon with Asparagus and Quinoa

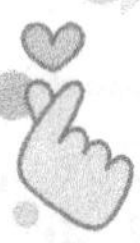

Procedure:

1. Preheat oven to 400°F. Line a baking sheet with parchment paper.

2. Place the salmon fillets and asparagus spears on the prepared baking sheet. Drizzle with 1 tbsp of the olive oil and season with salt and pepper.

3. Bake for 12•15 minutes, until the salmon is cooked through and the asparagus is tender.

4. In a small bowl, whisk together the remaining 1 tbsp olive oil, lemon juice, Dijon mustard, garlic, and dried dill. Season with salt and pepper.

5. Divide the cooked quinoa among 4 plates. Top each with a salmon fillet and some of the roasted asparagus spears.

6. Drizzle the lemon•Dijon dressing over the top.

Nutrition Info (per serving):
Calories: 350
Carbs: 20g
Fiber: 4g
Protein: 35g
Fat: 16g
Sodium: 350mg

This baked salmon dish is an excellent choice for a diabetic•friendly meal. Salmon is high in heart•healthy omega•3 fatty acids, while the quinoa and asparagus provide complex carbs, fiber, and important vitamins and minerals. The simple lemon•Dijon dressing adds flavor without adding too many calories or carbs.

You can adjust the portion sizes or swap in different vegetables to suit your preferences. !

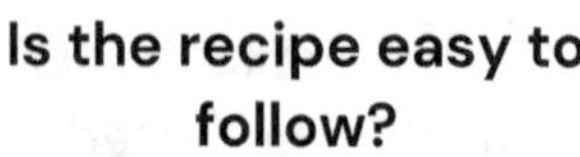

What is the total cooking time, including prep time?

Prep Time : ________________

Cook Time : ________________

Servings   : ________________

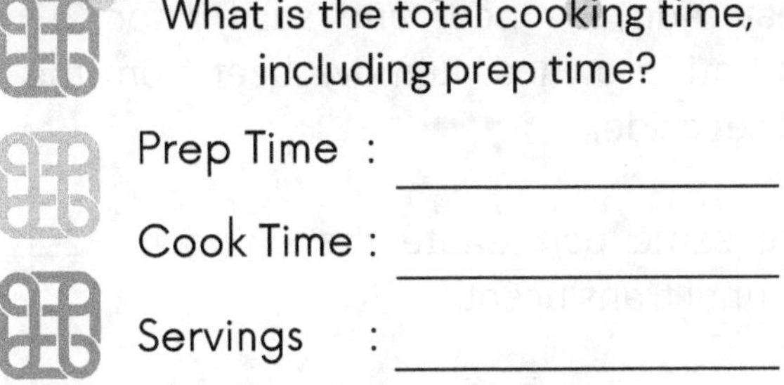

Ingredients:

For the Turkey Burgers:
• 1 lb ground turkey breast
• 1 egg white
• 1/4 cup whole wheat breadcrumbs
• 2 tbsp finely chopped onion
• 1 tsp Dijon mustard
• 1/2 tsp garlic powder
• 1/4 tsp salt
• 1/4 tsp black pepper

For the Sweet Potato Fries:
• 2 medium sweet potatoes, peeled and cut into 1/2•inch thick fries
• 1 tbsp olive oil
• 1/2 tsp paprika
• 1/4 tsp salt

To Serve:
• 4 whole wheat burger buns
• Lettuce, tomato, onion (optional toppings)

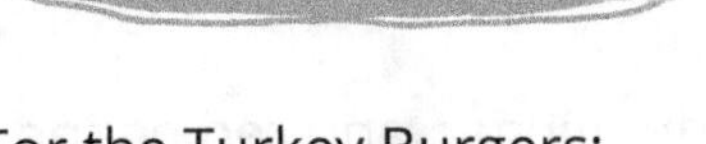

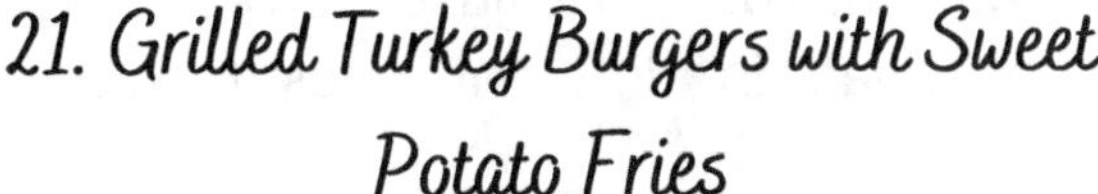

21. Grilled Turkey Burgers with Sweet Potato Fries

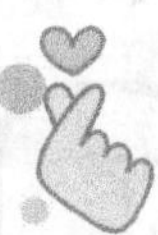

For the Turkey Burgers:
1. In a bowl, gently mix together all the burger ingredients until just combined. Form into 4 equal•sized patties.

2. Preheat grill or grill pan to medium•high heat. Cook the turkey burgers for 4•5 minutes per side, until cooked through.

For the Sweet Potato Fries:
1. Preheat oven to 400°F. Line a baking sheet with parchment paper.

2. Toss the sweet potato fries with the olive oil, paprika, and salt. Spread in a single layer on the prepared baking sheet.

3. Bake for 20•25 minutes, flipping halfway, until fries are tender and lightly browned.

To Serve:
1. Place each turkey burger on a whole wheat bun. Top with desired toppings.

2. Serve the sweet potato fries alongside the burgers.

Nutrition Info (per serving):
Calories: 400
Carbs: 40g
Fiber: 6g
Protein: 35g
Fat: 12g
Sodium: 550mg

This grilled turkey burger with sweet potato fries is a balanced, diabetic•friendly meal. The lean turkey patty provides protein, while the sweet potato fries are a healthier alternative to regular french fries. The whole wheat bun and toppings add fiber and nutrients. Adjust the portion sizes as needed.

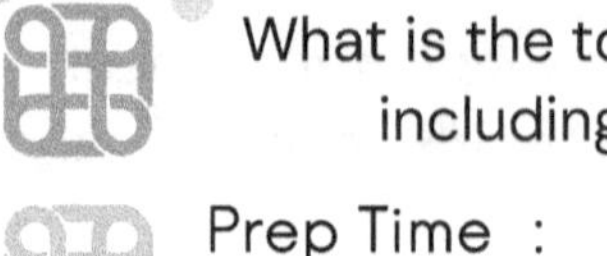

What are the critical points in the recipe (e.g., temperature control, timing)?

What is the total cooking time, including prep time?

Prep Time : _______________

Cook Time : _______________

Servings   : _______________

Ingredients:

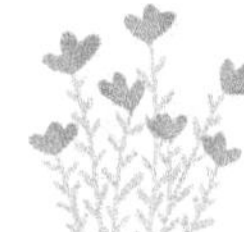

• 1 lb lean beef sirloin or flank steak, thinly sliced
• 2 tbsp low•sodium soy sauce
• 1 tbsp rice vinegar
• 1 tsp sesame oil
• 1 tsp cornstarch
• 2 cups cooked brown rice
• 2 tbsp olive oil
• 1 onion, sliced
• 2 cups broccoli florets
• 1 red bell pepper, sliced
• 2 cups sliced mushrooms
• 2 cloves garlic, minced
• 1 tsp grated fresh ginger
• 1/4 tsp red pepper flakes (optional)
• Salt and pepper to taste
• 2 tbsp chopped green onions (for garnish)

Is the recipe easy to follow?

22. Beef and Vegetable Stir•Fry with Brown Rice

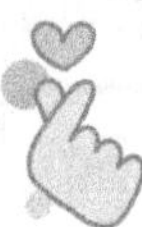

Procedure:

1. In a bowl, combine the sliced beef, soy sauce, rice vinegar, sesame oil, and cornstarch. Toss to coat the beef and let marinate for 15 minutes.

2. Heat the olive oil in a large skillet or wok over high heat. Add the beef and stir•fry for 2•3 minutes until browned. Remove beef from the pan and set aside.

3. In the same pan, sauté the onion for 2•3 minutes until translucent.

4. Add the broccoli, bell pepper, and mushrooms. Stir•fry for 4•5 minutes until vegetables are tender•crisp.

5. Stir in the garlic, ginger, and red pepper flakes (if using). Cook for 1 minute until fragrant.

6. Return the cooked beef to the pan and toss everything together. Season with salt and pepper.

7. Serve the beef and vegetable stir•fry over the cooked brown rice, garnished with chopped green onions.

Nutrition Info (per serving):
Calories: 400
Carbs: 35g
Fiber: 5g
Protein: 35g
Fat: 15g
Sodium: 450mg

This beef and vegetable stir•fry is a great diabetic•friendly meal. The lean beef provides protein, while the brown rice, vegetables, and Asian•inspired seasonings make it a balanced and flavorful dish. You can adjust the vegetable amounts or swap in different ones to your liking.

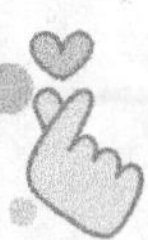

What are the critical points in the recipe (e.g., temperature control, timing)?

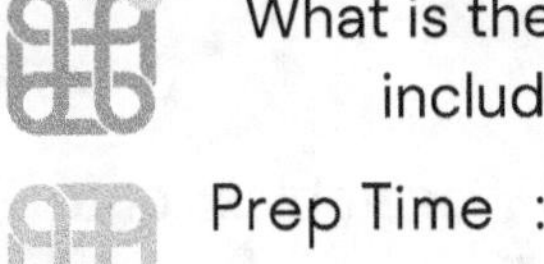

What is the total cooking time, including prep time?

Prep Time : ________________

Cook Time : ________________

Servings   : ________________

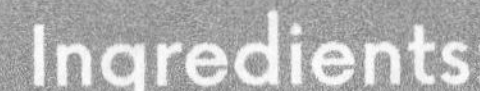 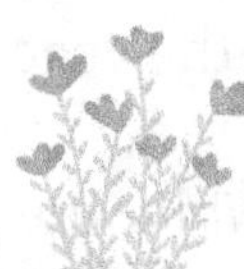

Ingredients:

• 4 medium zucchini, halved lengthwise
• 1 lb lean ground turkey
• 1 cup cooked quinoa
• 1/2 cup diced onion
• 2 cloves garlic, minced
• 1 tsp dried oregano
• 1/2 tsp dried basil
• 1/4 tsp red pepper flakes (optional)
• 1/2 cup shredded low•fat mozzarella cheese
• Salt and pepper to taste

Is the recipe easy to follow?

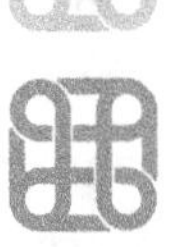

23. *Stuffed Zucchini Boats with Quinoa and Lean Turkey*

1. Preheat oven to 375°F. Spray a baking dish with non•stick cooking spray.

2. Scoop out the flesh from the zucchini halves, leaving about 1/4 inch of the zucchini shell. Finely chop the scooped out zucchini flesh.

3. In a skillet over medium heat, cook the ground turkey, chopped zucchini flesh, onion, and garlic until the turkey is browned and the vegetables are tender, about 5•7 minutes. Drain any excess fat.

4. Stir in the cooked quinoa, oregano, basil, and red pepper flakes (if using). Season with salt and pepper.

5. Arrange the zucchini boats in the prepared baking dish. Spoon the turkey•quinoa mixture evenly into the zucchini shells.

6. Top each stuffed zucchini boat with a sprinkle of shredded mozzarella cheese.

7. Bake for 20•25 minutes, until the zucchini is tender and the cheese is melted. Serve the stuffed zucchini boats warm.

Nutrition Info (per serving):
Calories: 250
Carbs: 18g
Fiber: 4g
Protein: 26g
Fat: 10g
Sodium: 350mg

These stuffed zucchini boats are a great diabetic•friendly meal. The lean turkey and quinoa provide protein and complex carbs, while the zucchini and other vegetables add fiber and nutrients. You can adjust the spices or add other veggies to your liking.

What is the total cooking time, including prep time?

Prep Time : ______________

Cook Time : ______________

Servings   : ______________

Ingredients:

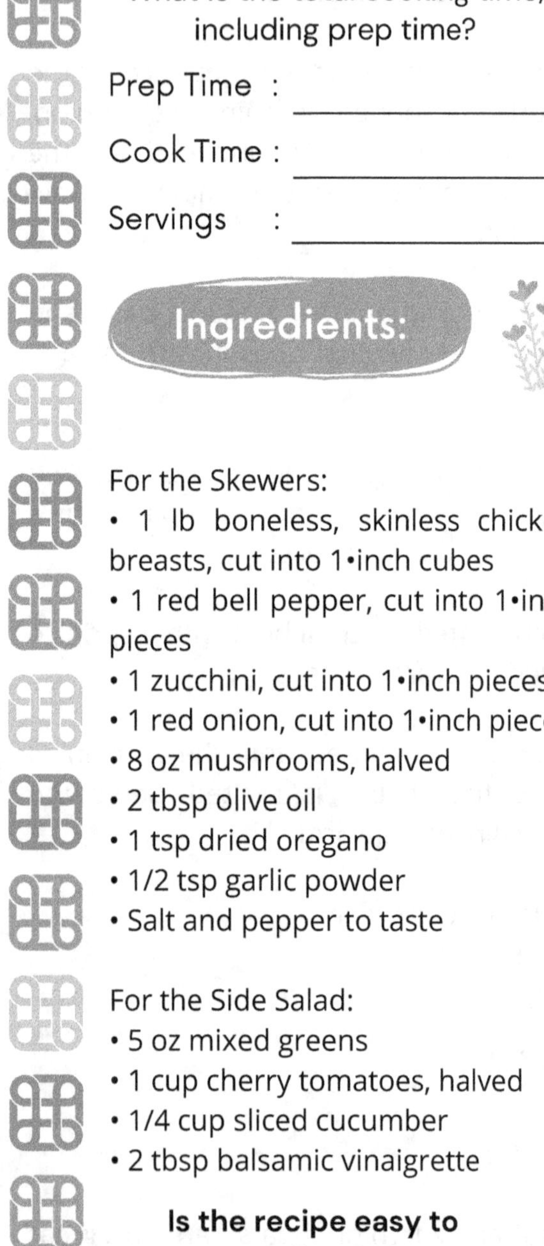

For the Skewers:
• 1 lb boneless, skinless chicken breasts, cut into 1·inch cubes
• 1 red bell pepper, cut into 1·inch pieces
• 1 zucchini, cut into 1·inch pieces
• 1 red onion, cut into 1·inch pieces
• 8 oz mushrooms, halved
• 2 tbsp olive oil
• 1 tsp dried oregano
• 1/2 tsp garlic powder
• Salt and pepper to taste

For the Side Salad:
• 5 oz mixed greens
• 1 cup cherry tomatoes, halved
• 1/4 cup sliced cucumber
• 2 tbsp balsamic vinaigrette

Is the recipe easy to follow?

24. Vegetable and Chicken Skewers with a Side Salad

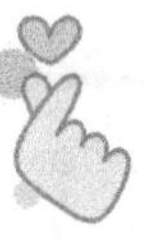

Procedure:

1. Preheat grill or grill pan to medium·high heat.

2. In a large bowl, toss the chicken, bell pepper, zucchini, onion, and mushrooms with the olive oil, oregano, garlic powder, salt, and pepper until evenly coated.

3. Thread the chicken and vegetables onto skewers, alternating the ingredients.

4. Grill the skewers for 12·15 minutes, turning occasionally, until the chicken is cooked through and the vegetables are tender.

5. While the skewers are cooking, prepare the side salad. In a large bowl, combine the mixed greens, cherry tomatoes, and cucumber. Drizzle with the balsamic vinaigrette and toss to coat.

6. Serve the grilled chicken and vegetable skewers alongside the side salad.

Nutrition Info (per serving):
Calories: 350
Carbs: 20g
Fiber: 5g
Protein: 35g
Fat: 15g
Sodium: 350mg

This meal of grilled chicken and vegetable skewers with a side salad is a great diabetic·friendly option. The lean protein from the chicken, fiber and nutrients from the vegetables, and healthy fats from the vinaigrette make it a balanced and satisfying meal. You can adjust the vegetable selection to your liking.

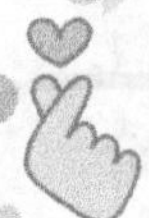

What are the critical points in the recipe (e.g., temperature control, timing)?

What is the total cooking time, including prep time?

Prep Time : ___________________

Cook Time : ___________________

Servings   : ___________________

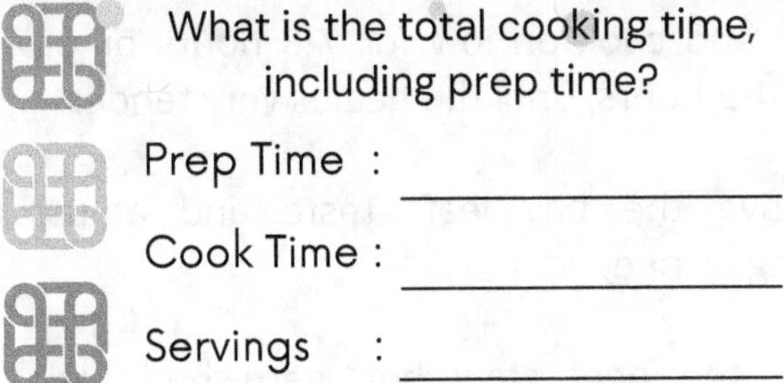

Ingredients:

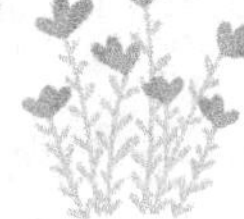

For the Cod:
- 4 (4 oz) cod fillets
- 1 tbsp olive oil
- 1 tbsp lemon juice
- 1 tsp dried parsley
- 1/4 tsp garlic powder
- Salt and pepper to taste

For the Quinoa:
- 1 cup cooked quinoa
- 2 tbsp chopped fresh parsley
- 2 tbsp chopped fresh dill
- 1 tbsp lemon juice
- 1 tsp lemon zest
- 1 tbsp olive oil
- Salt and pepper to taste

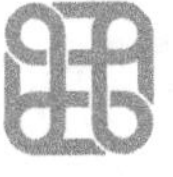

Is the recipe easy to follow?

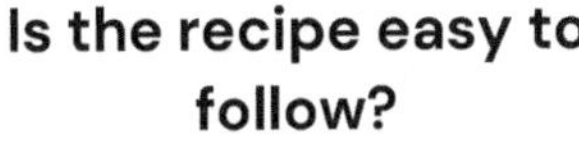

25. Baked Cod with Lemon and Herb Quinoa

1. Preheat oven to 400°F. Line a baking sheet with parchment paper.

2. Place the cod fillets on the prepared baking sheet. Drizzle with the olive oil and lemon juice, then sprinkle with the dried parsley, garlic powder, salt, and pepper.

3. Bake the cod for 12•15 minutes, until it flakes easily with a fork.

4. While the cod is baking, prepare the lemon and herb quinoa. In a medium bowl, combine the cooked quinoa, fresh parsley, dill, lemon juice, lemon zest, olive oil, salt, and pepper. Stir to mix well.

5. Serve the baked cod fillets over the lemon and herb quinoa.

Nutrition Info (per serving):
Calories: 320
Carbs: 25g
Fiber: 4g
Protein: 35g
Fat: 12g
Sodium: 350mg

This baked cod with lemon and herb quinoa is an excellent diabetic•friendly meal. The cod provides lean protein, while the quinoa offers complex carbs and fiber. The fresh herbs and lemon add lots of flavor without adding many calories or carbs.

You can adjust the portion sizes or swap In different herbs to your liking. This makes a balanced, nutrient•dense meal that is perfect for seniors with diabetes.

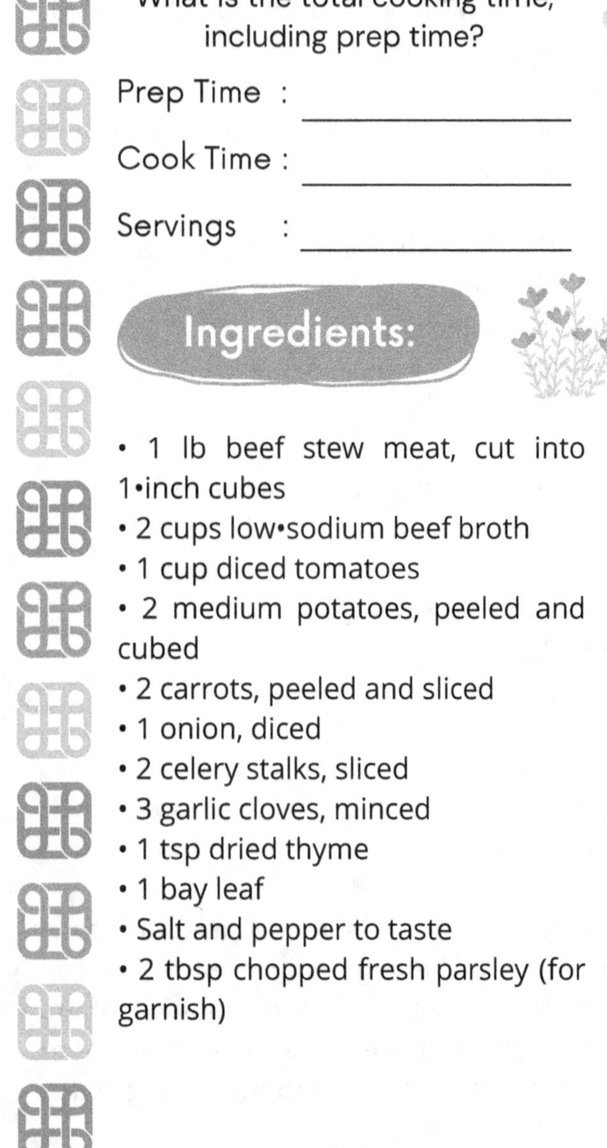

What are the critical points in the recipe (e.g., temperature control, timing)?

What is the total cooking time, including prep time?

Prep Time : _______________

Cook Time : _______________

Servings   : _______________

- 1 lb beef stew meat, cut into 1·inch cubes
- 2 cups low·sodium beef broth
- 1 cup diced tomatoes
- 2 medium potatoes, peeled and cubed
- 2 carrots, peeled and sliced
- 1 onion, diced
- 2 celery stalks, sliced
- 3 garlic cloves, minced
- 1 tsp dried thyme
- 1 bay leaf
- Salt and pepper to taste
- 2 tbsp chopped fresh parsley (for garnish)

Is the recipe easy to follow?

☺   ☹

26. Slow·Cooked Beef Stew with Vegetables

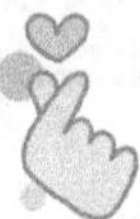

1. In a slow cooker, combine the beef, beef broth, diced tomatoes, potatoes, carrots, onion, celery, garlic, thyme, and bay leaf. Season with salt and pepper.

2. Cover and cook on low for 7·8 hours or on high for 4·5 hours, until the beef is very tender.

3. Remove the bay leaf. Taste and adjust seasoning as needed.

4. Serve the beef stew hot, garnished with chopped fresh parsley.

Nutrition Info (per serving):
Calories: 300
Carbs: 25g
Fiber: 5g
Protein: 30g
Fat: 8g
Sodium: 350mg

This slow·cooked beef stew is a great diabetic·friendly meal. The lean beef provides protein, while the vegetables add fiber, vitamins, and minerals. The long cooking time helps tenderize the meat and allows the flavors to meld together.

You can serve this stew on its own or with a side of whole grain bread or brown rice. Adjust the vegetable amounts to your liking. The slow cooker makes this an easy, hands·off meal.

!

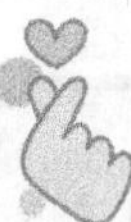

What are the critical points in the recipe (e.g., temperature control, timing)?

What is the total cooking time, including prep time?

Prep Time : ________________

Cook Time : ________________

Servings   : ________________

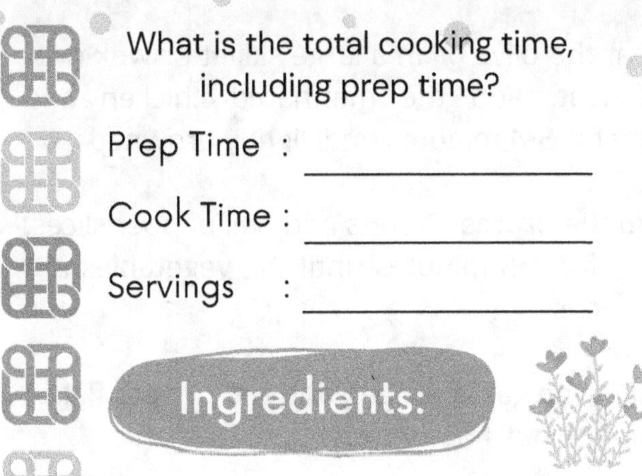

Ingredients:

For the Shrimp:
• 1 lb large shrimp, peeled and deveined
• 1 tbsp olive oil
• 1 tsp lemon juice
• 1 tsp dried oregano
• 1/4 tsp garlic powder
• Salt and pepper to taste

For the Spinach Salad:
• 5 oz baby spinach
• 1 cup cherry tomatoes, halved
• 1/2 cucumber, sliced
• 2 tbsp crumbled feta cheese
• 2 tbsp balsamic vinaigrette

Is the recipe easy to follow?

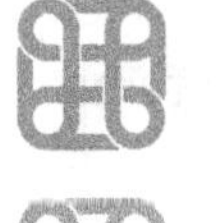

27. Grilled Shrimp with a Spinach Salad

1. Preheat grill or grill pan to medium•high heat.

2. In a bowl, toss the shrimp with the olive oil, lemon juice, oregano, garlic powder, salt, and pepper.

3. Thread the seasoned shrimp onto skewers.

4. Grill the shrimp skewers for 2•3 minutes per side, until the shrimp are opaque and cooked through.

5. In a large salad bowl, combine the baby spinach, cherry tomatoes, cucumber, and feta cheese.

6. Drizzle the balsamic vinaigrette over the salad and toss gently to coat.

7. Serve the grilled shrimp skewers alongside the spinach salad.

Nutrition Info (per serving):
Calories: 300
Carbs: 15g
Fiber: 4g
Protein: 30g
Fat: 12g
Sodium: 450mg

This grilled shrimp with spinach salad is an excellent diabetic•friendly meal. The shrimp provides lean protein, while the spinach, tomatoes, and cucumber in the salad offer fiber, vitamins, and minerals. The balsamic vinaigrette adds flavor without too many carbs.

You can adjust the portion sizes or swap in different greens or vegetables in the salad to your liking. This makes a light, yet satisfying and nutritious meal.

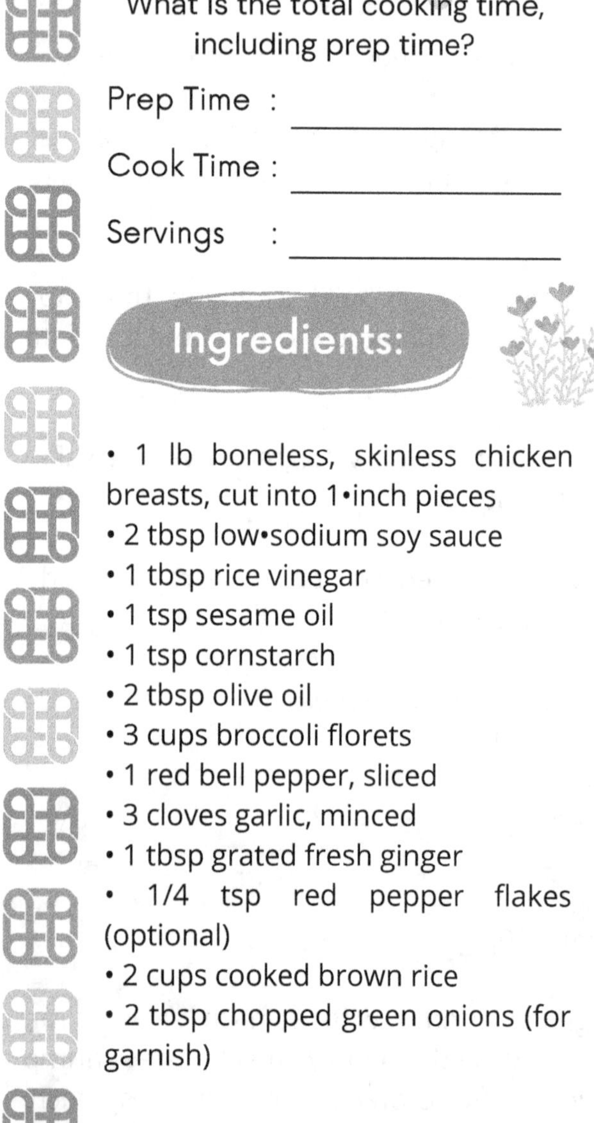

What is the total cooking time, including prep time?

Prep Time : _______________

Cook Time : _______________

Servings : _______________

Ingredients:

• 1 lb boneless, skinless chicken breasts, cut into 1•inch pieces
• 2 tbsp low•sodium soy sauce
• 1 tbsp rice vinegar
• 1 tsp sesame oil
• 1 tsp cornstarch
• 2 tbsp olive oil
• 3 cups broccoli florets
• 1 red bell pepper, sliced
• 3 cloves garlic, minced
• 1 tbsp grated fresh ginger
• 1/4 tsp red pepper flakes (optional)
• 2 cups cooked brown rice
• 2 tbsp chopped green onions (for garnish)

Is the recipe easy to follow?

🙂   🙁

28. Chicken and Broccoli Stir•Fry

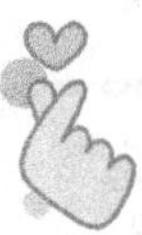

Procedure:

1. In a bowl, combine the chicken, soy sauce, rice vinegar, sesame oil, and cornstarch. Toss to coat the chicken and let marinate for 15 minutes.

2. Heat the olive oil in a large skillet or wok over high heat. Add the marinated chicken and stir•fry for 3•4 minutes until lightly browned.

3. Add the broccoli florets and bell pepper slices. Stir•fry for 4•5 minutes until the vegetables are tender•crisp.

4. Stir in the garlic, ginger, and red pepper flakes (if using). Cook for 1 minute until fragrant.

5. Serve the chicken and broccoli stir•fry over the cooked brown rice, garnished with chopped green onions.

Nutrition Info (per serving):
Calories: 350
Carbs: 35g
Fiber: 5g
Protein: 35g
Fat: 10g
Sodium: 450mg

This chicken and broccoli stir•fry is a great diabetic•friendly meal. The lean chicken provides protein, while the broccoli and brown rice offer fiber and complex carbs. The Asian•inspired flavors from the soy sauce, ginger, and garlic make it a tasty and satisfying dish.

You can adjust the vegetable amounts or swap in different ones to your liking. Serve it with a side salad for an even more well•rounded meal.

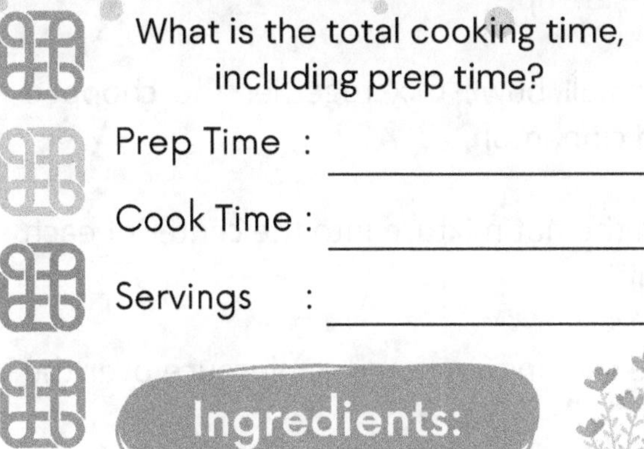

What is the total cooking time, including prep time?

Prep Time : ___________________

Cook Time : ___________________

Servings   : ___________________

Ingredients:

- 1/4 cup chia seeds
- 1 cup unsweetened almond milk
- 1 tsp vanilla extract
- 1/2 tsp ground cinnamon
- 1 tbsp honey (optional)
- 1 cup fresh berries (such as raspberries, blueberries, or strawberries)

Is the recipe easy to follow?

29. Chia Pudding with Fresh Berries

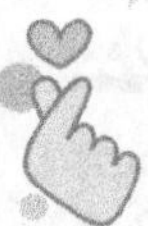

Procedure:

1. In a medium bowl, whisk together the chia seeds, almond milk, vanilla, and cinnamon until well combined.

2. Cover the bowl and refrigerate for at least 2 hours, or overnight, stirring occasionally, until the chia pudding has thickened.

3. If using honey, stir it into the chia pudding just before serving.

4. Divide the chia pudding into 2 serving bowls or glasses.

5. Top each serving with 1/2 cup of fresh berries.

This chia pudding with fresh berries is an excellent diabetic-friendly snack or dessert. Here's why:

- Chia seeds are high in fiber, protein, and healthy fats, which help stabilize blood sugar levels.

- Unsweetened almond milk is low in carbs and calories compared to dairy milk.

- Fresh berries provide natural sweetness along with antioxidants, vitamins, and minerals.

- The optional honey adds a touch of sweetness, but can be omitted if desired.

The combination of the nutrient-dense chia pudding and fresh berries makes this a satisfying and diabetes-friendly treat. You can adjust the amount of honey or try different types of berries to suit your taste preferences.

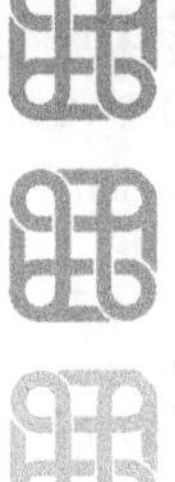
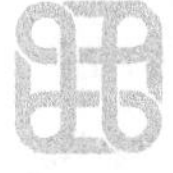
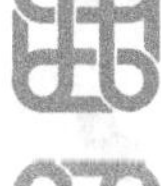
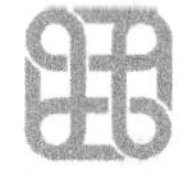

What are the critical points in the recipe (e.g., temperature control, timing)?

What is the total cooking time, including prep time?

Prep Time : ______________

Cook Time : ______________

Servings   : ______________

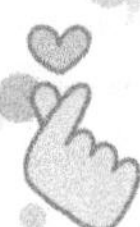

Ingredients:

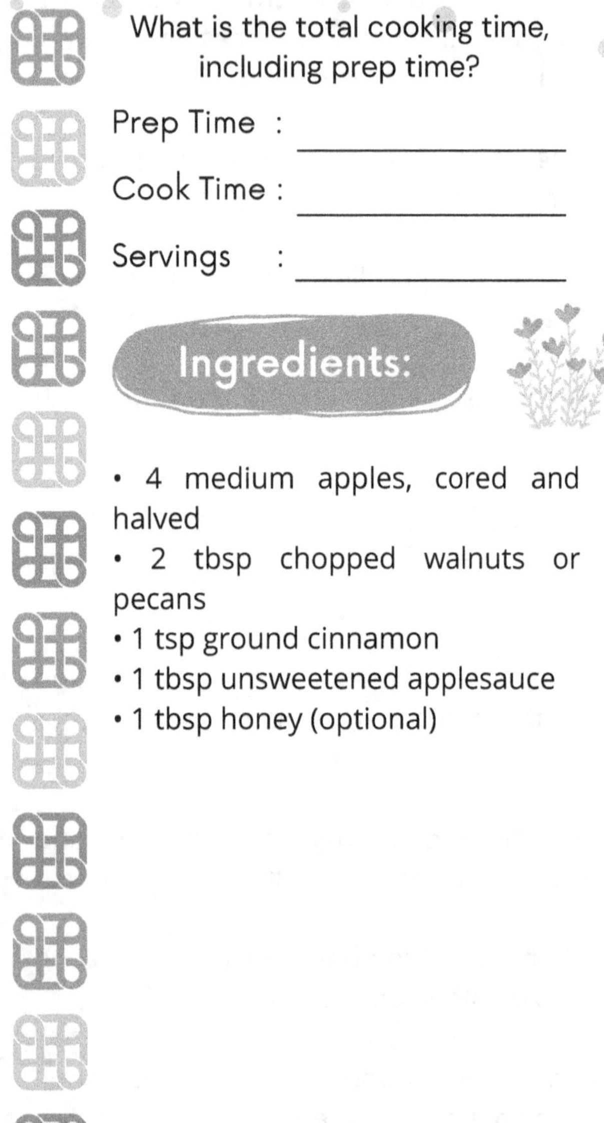

- 4 medium apples, cored and halved
- 2 tbsp chopped walnuts or pecans
- 1 tsp ground cinnamon
- 1 tbsp unsweetened applesauce
- 1 tbsp honey (optional)

Is the recipe easy to follow?

30. Baked Apples with Cinnamon and Nuts

Procedure:

1. Preheat oven to 375°F. Lightly grease a baking dish.

2. Place the apple halves in the prepared baking dish, cut•side up.

3. In a small bowl, mix together the chopped nuts and cinnamon.

4. Spoon the nut mixture into the center of each apple half.

5. Drizzle the unsweetened applesauce over the apples.

6. If desired, drizzle a small amount of honey over the apples as well.

7. Bake for 20•25 minutes, until the apples are tender when pierced with a fork.

8. Serve the baked apples warm.

These baked apples make a great diabetic•friendly dessert. The apples provide natural sweetness, while the nuts add healthy fats and fiber to help slow the absorption of the carbs. The cinnamon also helps regulate blood sugar levels.

The unsweetened applesauce and optional honey provide just a touch of sweetness without spiking blood sugar too much. This makes a satisfying and nutritious treat.

You can adjust the amount of nuts or honey to your taste preferences. Enjoy these baked apples on their own or with a dollop of plain Greek yogurt.

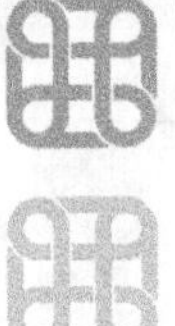

What are the critical points in the recipe (e.g., temperature control, timing)?

What is the total cooking time, including prep time?

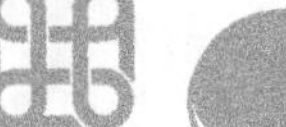

Prep Time : _______________

Cook Time : _______________

Servings : _______________

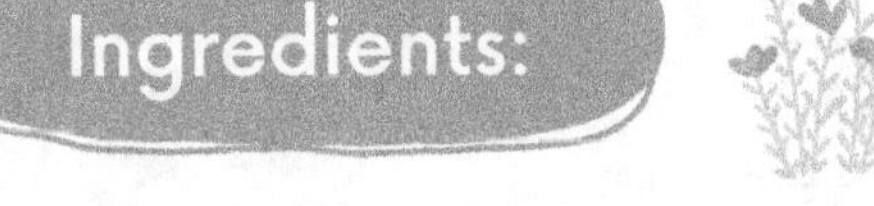

Ingredients:

• 1 cup plain, unsweetened Greek yogurt
• 1 tbsp raw, unprocessed honey
• 2 tbsp raw, unsalted almonds, chopped

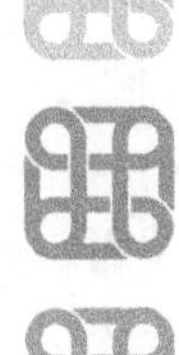
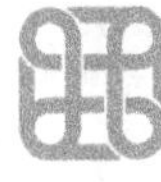
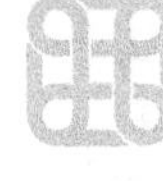
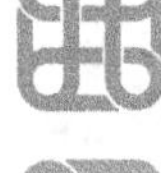
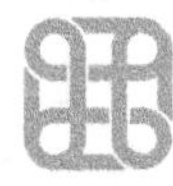

Is the recipe easy to follow?

31. *Greek Yogurt with Honey and Almonds*

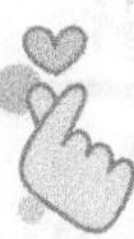

Procedure:

1. Scoop the Greek yogurt into a bowl.

2. Drizzle the honey over the yogurt.

3. Sprinkle the chopped almonds on top.

4. Stir everything together gently until well combined.

Nutrition Info (per serving):
Calories: 200
Carbs: 16g
Fiber: 3g
Protein: 18g
Fat: 9g
Net Carbs: 13g

This Greek yogurt with honey and almonds makes a great diabetic•friendly snack for a few reasons:

• Greek yogurt is high in protein, which helps stabilize blood sugar levels. Look for plain, unsweetened varieties.

• Honey provides a natural sweetness, but in moderation as it is still a carbohydrate. 1 tbsp is a good portion size.

• Almonds add healthy fats, fiber, and protein to help provide satiety and slow the absorption of the carbs.

The combination of the protein•rich yogurt, natural sweetener, and crunchy almonds makes this a balanced and satisfying snack option for those with diabetes. You can adjust the amounts to your taste preferences, but be mindful of the carb and calorie content.

!

What are the critical points in the recipe (e.g., temperature control, timing)?

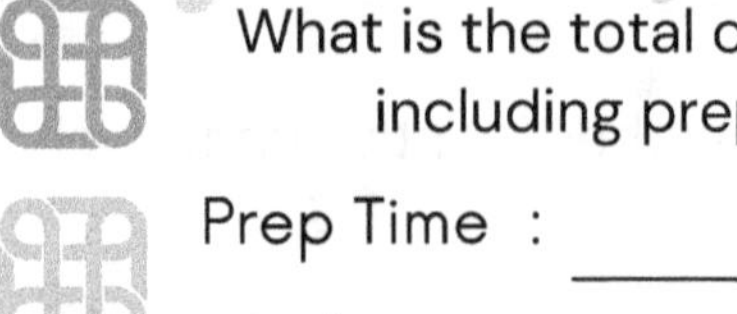

What is the total cooking time, including prep time?

Prep Time : ______________

Cook Time : ______________

Servings   : ______________

Ingredients:

• 1 oz dark chocolate (70% cacao or higher)
• 1 tbsp raw, unsalted almonds

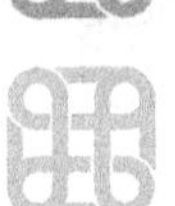

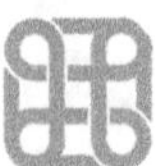
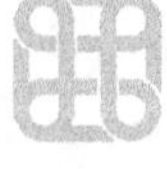
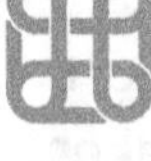
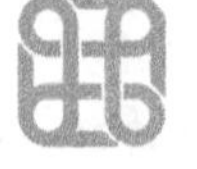

Is the recipe easy to follow?

32. Dark Chocolate with Almonds

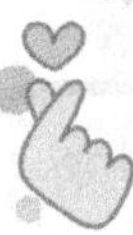

Procedure:

1. Break or chop the dark chocolate into small pieces.

2. Place the chocolate pieces and almonds in a small bowl.

Dark chocolate and almonds make a great diabetic·friendly snack for a few reasons:

Nutrition Info (per serving):
Calories: 150
Carbs: 10g
Fiber: 4g
Protein: 4g
Fat: 12g
Net Carbs: 6g

• Dark chocolate is high in antioxidants and has a lower sugar content compared to milk chocolate. The 70% cacao or higher provides more beneficial compounds.

• Almonds are a great source of healthy fats, fiber, and protein. They help provide satiety and stabilize blood sugar levels.

• The combination of the dark chocolate and almonds provides a satisfying sweet and crunchy snack.

This portion size of 1 oz dark chocolate and 1 tbsp almonds is a good balance for a diabetic·friendly treat. You can adjust the amounts to your preference, but be mindful of the carb and calorie content. Enjoy this snack in moderation as part of a healthy diabetic diet.

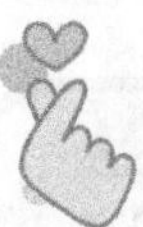

Procedure:

What is the total cooking time,
including prep time?

Prep Time   : ______________

Cook Time : ______________

Servings   : ______________

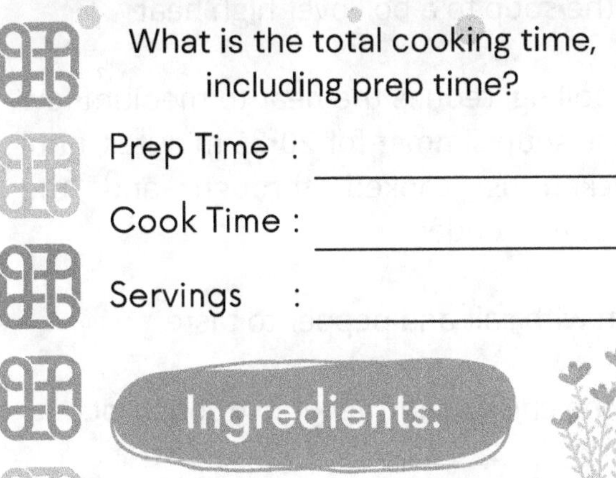

Ingredients:

• 1 cup plain, unsweetened Greek yogurt
• 1/2 cup mixed berries (such as raspberries, blueberries, and blackberries)
• 1 tbsp chopped walnuts or sliced almonds
• 1 tsp honey (optional)

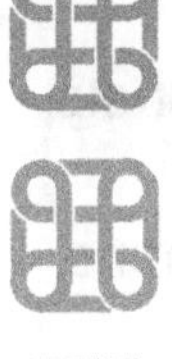
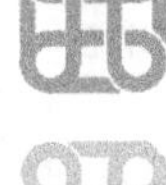
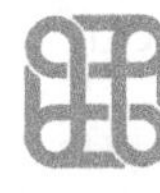
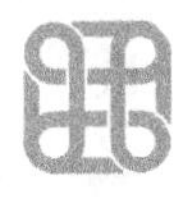

Is the recipe easy to follow?

33. *Mixed Berry Parfait with Greek Yogurt*

1. In a parfait glass or small bowl, layer half of the Greek yogurt.

2. Top the yogurt with half of the mixed berries.

3. Sprinkle half of the chopped nuts over the berries.

4. Repeat the layers, ending with the remaining yogurt, berries, and nuts.

5. If desired, drizzle the honey over the top of the parfait.

Nutrition Info (per serving):
Calories: 200
Carbs: 16g
Fiber: 5g
Protein: 18g
Fat: 9g
Net Carbs: 11g

This mixed berry parfait is a great diabetic•friendly dessert or snack:

• Greek yogurt is high in protein, which helps stabilize blood sugar levels.
• Mixed berries provide natural sweetness, fiber, and antioxidants.
• Nuts add healthy fats and a crunchy texture.
• The optional honey provides a touch of sweetness, but can be omitted.

The combination of the creamy yogurt, juicy berries, and crunchy nuts makes this parfait both satisfying and nutritious. You can adjust the amounts of each ingredient to suit your taste preferences.

This makes a great grab•and•go snack or a light, healthy dessert. Enjoy it as part of a balanced diabetic diet.

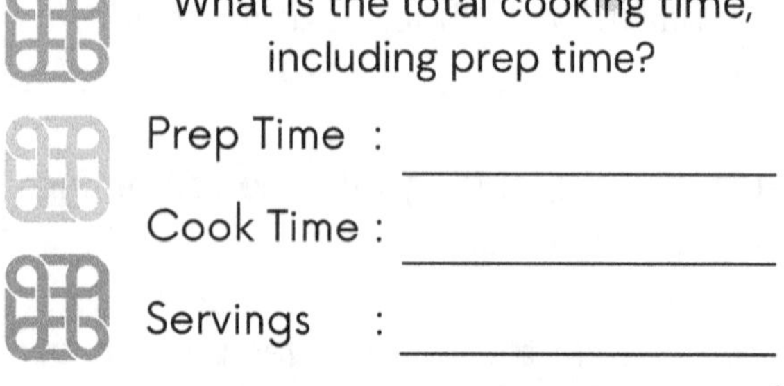

What are the critical points in the recipe (e.g., temperature control, timing)?

What is the total cooking time, including prep time?

Prep Time : _______________

Cook Time : _______________

Servings : _______________

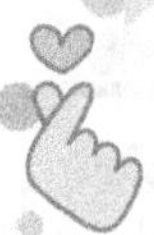

Ingredients:

- 1 lb boneless, skinless chicken breasts, cubed
- 4 cups low•sodium chicken broth
- 2 cups diced mixed vegetables (such as carrots, celery, onions, and zucchini)
- 1 cup chopped kale or spinach
- 1 tsp dried thyme
- 1 tsp dried parsley
- 1/2 tsp garlic powder
- Salt and pepper to taste

Is the recipe easy to follow?

34. Chicken and Vegetable Soup

1. In a large pot or Dutch oven, combine the cubed chicken, chicken broth, diced vegetables, kale/spinach, thyme, parsley, and garlic powder.

2. Bring the soup to a boil over high heat.

3. Once boiling, reduce the heat to medium•low and let the soup simmer for 20•25 minutes, until the chicken is cooked through and the vegetables are tender.

4. Season with salt and pepper to taste.

5. Serve the chicken and vegetable soup hot.

Nutrition Info (per serving):
Calories: 200
Carbs: 10g
Fiber: 3g
Protein: 30g
Fat: 3g
Sodium: 350mg

This chicken and vegetable soup is an excellent diabetic•friendly meal for a few reasons:

- Lean chicken breast provides protein to help stabilize blood sugar.
- The variety of vegetables add fiber, vitamins, and minerals.
- The low•sodium broth keeps the sodium content in check.
- The simple seasoning adds flavor without added sugars or fats.

This soup is easy to make and very versatile. You can adjust the vegetable selection based on your preferences. Serve it on its own or with a side salad or whole grain crackers for a complete and balanced meal.

!

What are the critical points in the recipe (e.g., temperature control, timing)?

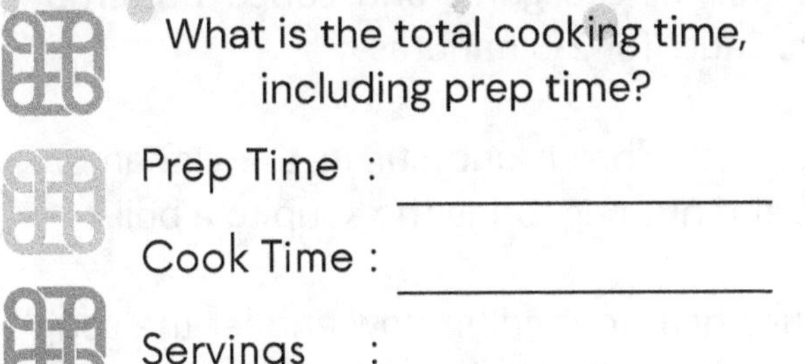

What is the total cooking time, including prep time?

Prep Time : _______________

Cook Time : _______________

Servings   : _______________

Ingredients:

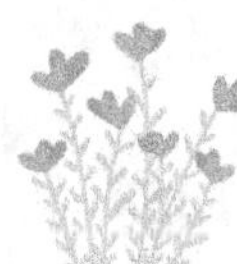

- 1 tbsp olive oil
- 1 onion, diced
- 2 carrots, peeled and diced
- 2 celery stalks, diced
- 3 cloves garlic, minced
- 1 (15 oz) can diced tomatoes
- 4 cups low·sodium vegetable or chicken broth
- 1 (15 oz) can kidney beans, rinsed and drained
- 1 cup chopped zucchini
- 1 cup frozen green beans
- 1 cup small whole wheat pasta (such as ditalini or elbow macaroni)
- 2 tsp dried Italian seasoning
- Salt and pepper to taste
- 2 tbsp grated Parmesan cheese (optional)

Is the recipe easy to follow?

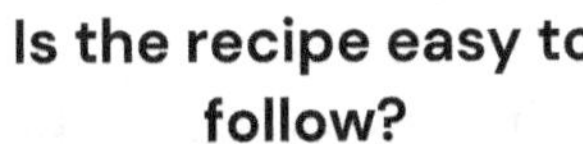

35. Minestrone Soup

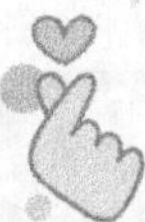

Procedure:

1. In a large pot, heat the olive oil over medium heat. Add the onion, carrots, celery, and garlic. Sauté for 5·7 minutes until the vegetables are softened.

2. Stir in the diced tomatoes, broth, kidney beans, zucchini, green beans, pasta, and Italian seasoning.

3. Bring the soup to a boil, then reduce heat and let simmer for 15·20 minutes, until the pasta is tender.

4. Season with salt and pepper to taste. Serve the minestrone soup hot, garnished with grated Parmesan cheese if desired.

Nutrition Info (per serving):
Calories: 250
Carbs: 35g
Fiber: 8g
Protein: 12g
Fat: 6g
Sodium: 450mg

This minestrone soup is an excellent diabetic·friendly meal for several reasons:

- The variety of vegetables provide fiber, vitamins, and minerals.
- The beans add protein and complex carbs to help stabilize blood sugar.
- The whole wheat pasta offers more fiber than regular pasta.
- The low·sodium broth keeps the sodium content in check.

This hearty soup is easy to make and very versatile. You can adjust the vegetable selection or add other beans to your liking. Serve it with a side salad or some whole grain bread for a complete and balanced meal.

What is the total cooking time, including prep time?

Prep Time : _______________

Cook Time : _______________

Servings : _______________

Ingredients:

- 1 medium butternut squash, peeled, seeded, and cubed (about 4 cups)
- 1 tbsp olive oil
- 1 onion, diced
- 2 cloves garlic, minced
- 4 cups low•sodium chicken or vegetable broth
- 1 tsp ground cinnamon
- 1/2 tsp ground ginger
- 1/4 tsp ground nutmeg
- Salt and pepper to taste
- 2 tbsp plain Greek yogurt (optional garnish)
- 2 tbsp chopped toasted walnuts (optional garnish)

Is the recipe easy to follow?

36. Butternut Squash Soup

Procedure:

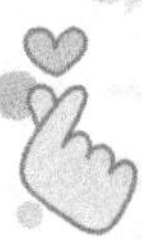

1. In a large pot or Dutch oven, heat the olive oil over medium heat. Add the diced onion and sauté for 3•4 minutes until translucent.

2. Add the minced garlic and cubed butternut squash. Sauté for 2•3 minutes.

3. Pour in the broth and stir in the cinnamon, ginger, and nutmeg. Bring the soup to a boil.

4. Reduce heat to medium•low and let the soup simmer for 20•25 minutes, until the squash is very soft.

5. Using an immersion blender or regular blender, puree the soup until smooth.

6. Season with salt and pepper to taste.

7. Serve the butternut squash soup warm, garnished with a dollop of Greek yogurt and chopped toasted walnuts if desired.

This butternut squash soup is an excellent diabetic•friendly option for several reasons:

- Butternut squash is high in fiber, vitamins, and complex carbs.
- The broth keeps the soup light and low in calories.
- The warming spices like cinnamon and ginger can help regulate blood sugar.
- The optional Greek yogurt and walnuts add protein and healthy fats.

This soup is easy to make and very comforting. Adjust the seasoning to your taste preferences. Serve it as a starter or pair it with a salad or whole grain bread for a complete meal.

What are the critical points in the recipe (e.g., temperature control, timing)?

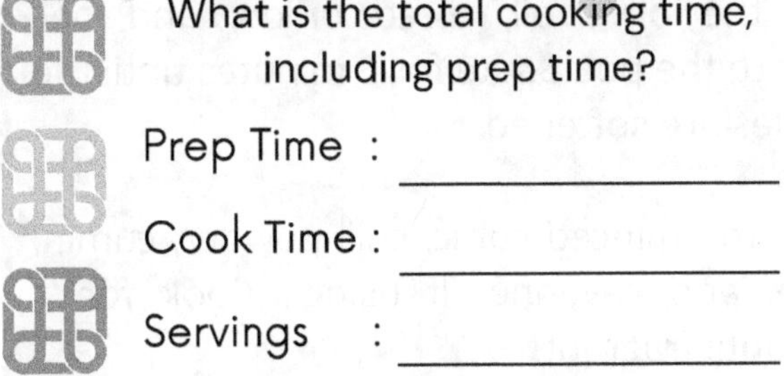

What is the total cooking time, including prep time?

Prep Time : ________________

Cook Time : ________________

Servings   : ________________

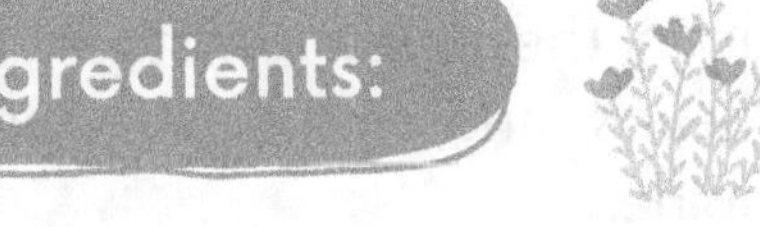

Ingredients:

- 1 lb lean beef stew meat, cut into 1•inch cubes
- 2 tbsp olive oil
- 1 onion, diced
- 2 carrots, peeled and diced
- 2 celery stalks, diced
- 3 cloves garlic, minced
- 4 cups low•sodium beef broth
- 1 cup pearl barley
- 1 (14.5 oz) can diced tomatoes
- 2 tsp dried thyme
- 1 bay leaf
- Salt and pepper to taste
- 2 tbsp chopped fresh parsley (for garnish)

Is the recipe easy to follow?

37. Beef and Barley Stew

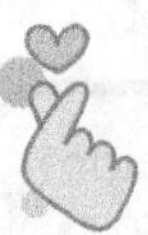

Procedure:

1. In a large pot or Dutch oven, heat the olive oil over medium•high heat. Add the beef cubes and brown on all sides, about 3•4 minutes per side. Remove beef from the pot and set aside.

2. Add the diced onion, carrots, and celery to the pot. Sauté for 5•7 minutes until the vegetables are softened.

3. Stir in the minced garlic and cook for 1 minute until fragrant.

4. Pour in the beef broth and add the pearl barley, diced tomatoes, thyme, and bay leaf.

5. Return the browned beef to the pot and bring the stew to a boil.

6. Reduce heat to medium•low, cover, and let the stew simmer for 45•60 minutes, until the beef is very tender and the barley is cooked through.

7. Season with salt and pepper to taste. Serve the beef and barley stew hot, garnished with chopped fresh parsley.

This beef and barley stew is an excellent diabetic•friendly meal for several reasons:

- Lean beef provides protein to help stabilize blood sugar.
- Pearl barley is a whole grain that is high in fiber.
- The vegetables add nutrients and fiber.

The combination of the tender beef, hearty barley, and nutrient•dense vegetables makes this stew very satisfying and nutritious. Adjust the vegetable amounts to your liking. Serve it on its own or with a side salad for a complete meal.

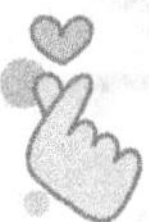

What are the critical points in the recipe (e.g., temperature control, timing)?

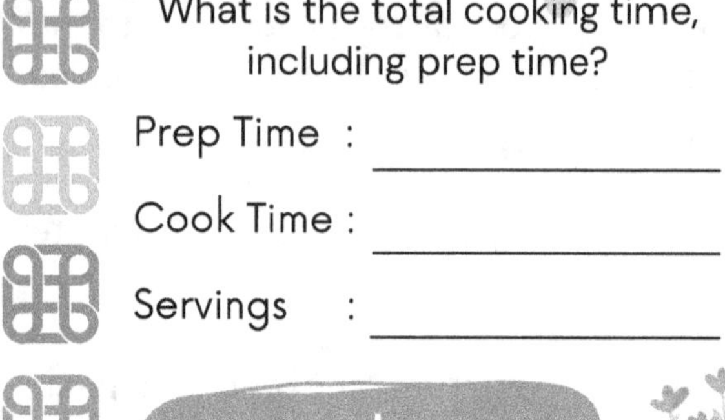

What is the total cooking time, including prep time?

Prep Time : _______________

Cook Time : _______________

Servings   : _______________

Ingredients:

- 1 lb ground turkey
- 1 tbsp olive oil
- 1 onion, diced
- 2 bell peppers, diced
- 3 cloves garlic, minced
- 2 tbsp chili powder
- 1 tsp ground cumin
- 1 tsp dried oregano
- 1/4 tsp cayenne pepper (optional)
- 1 (15 oz) can diced tomatoes
- 1 (15 oz) can kidney beans, rinsed and drained
- 1 (15 oz) can black beans, rinsed and drained
- 1 cup low•sodium chicken or vegetable broth
- Salt and pepper to taste
- 2 tbsp chopped fresh cilantro (for garnish)

Is the recipe easy to follow?

38. Turkey and Bean Chili

Procedure:

1. In a large pot or Dutch oven, cook the ground turkey over medium•high heat, breaking it up with a wooden spoon, until browned, about 5•7 minutes. Drain any excess fat.

2. Add the olive oil, diced onion, and bell peppers to the pot. Sauté for 5 minutes until the vegetables are softened.

3. Stir in the minced garlic, chili powder, cumin, oregano, and cayenne (if using). Cook for 1 minute until fragrant.

4. Pour in the diced tomatoes, kidney beans, black beans, and chicken/vegetable broth. Stir to combine.

5. Bring the chili to a boil, then reduce heat and let it simmer for 20•25 minutes, stirring occasionally, until thickened.

6. Season with salt and pepper to taste. Serve the turkey and bean chili hot, garnished with chopped fresh cilantro.

This turkey and bean chili is an excellent diabetic•friendly meal for several reasons:

- Ground turkey is a lean protein that won't spike blood sugar.
- Beans provide fiber and complex carbs to help stabilize blood sugar.
- The vegetables add nutrients and fiber.
- The spices provide flavor without added sugars.

The combination of the protein, fiber, and complex carbs makes this chili very satisfying and nutritious. You can adjust the spice level to your preferences. Serve it on its own or with a side salad for a complete meal.

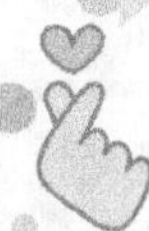

Procedure:

1. In a large pot, combine the lentils and vegetable broth. Bring to a boil, then reduce heat and simmer for 15•20 minutes, until lentils are tender.

2. In a large skillet, heat the olive oil over medium heat. Add the onion and sauté for 5 minutes until translucent.

3. Add the garlic, carrots, celery and bell pepper. Sauté for 5•7 minutes until vegetables are starting to soften.

4. Add the diced tomatoes, thyme, oregano, smoked paprika, salt and pepper. Stir to combine.

5. Add the cooked lentils and vegetable broth to the skillet. Bring to a simmer and cook for 10•15 minutes, until vegetables are tender.

6. Taste and adjust seasonings as needed. Serve hot, garnished with chopped parsley if desired.

Enjoy your hearty and nutritious Vegetable Lentil Stew!

What is the total cooking time, including prep time?

Prep Time : _______________

Cook Time : _______________

Servings   : _______________

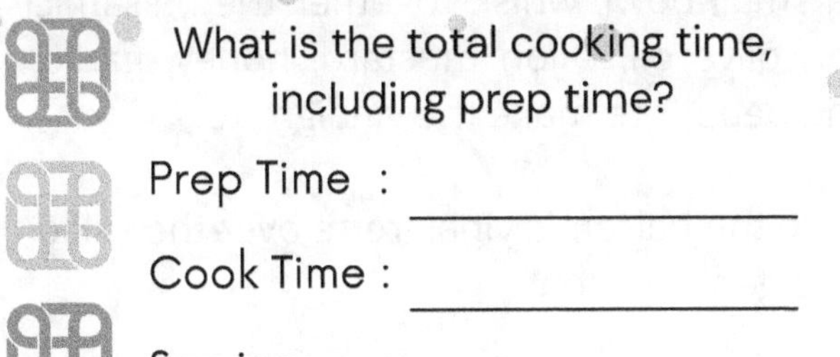

Ingredients:

• 1 cup dry brown or green lentils, rinsed
• 4 cups vegetable broth
• 1 tablespoon olive oil
• 1 onion, diced
• 3 cloves garlic, minced
• 2 carrots, peeled and diced
• 2 celery stalks, diced
• 1 red bell pepper, diced
• 1 (14.5 oz) can diced tomatoes
• 2 teaspoons dried thyme
• 1 teaspoon dried oregano
• 1/2 teaspoon smoked paprika
• Salt and black pepper to taste
• Chopped parsley for garnish (optional)

Is the recipe easy to follow?

39. Vegetable Lentil Stew

What is the total cooking time, including prep time?

Prep Time : ___________________

Cook Time : ___________________

Servings : ___________________

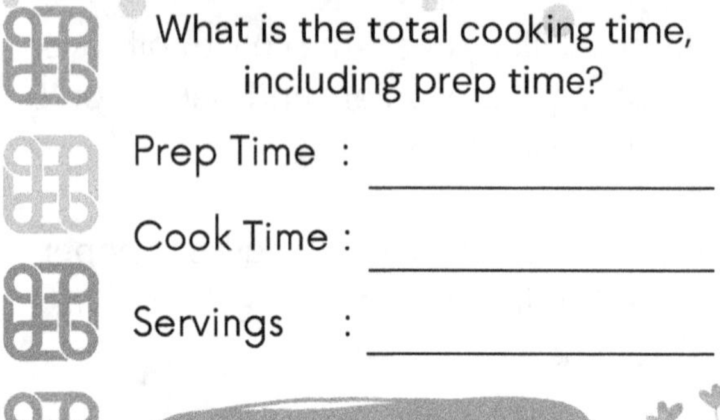

Ingredients:

• 6 cups mixed greens (such as spinach, arugula, kale, romaine)
• 1 cup cherry tomatoes, halved
• 1/2 cup sliced cucumber
• 1/4 cup sliced red onion
• 2 tablespoons crumbled feta cheese
• 2 tablespoons toasted slivered almonds

Balsamic Vinaigrette:
• 2 tablespoons balsamic vinegar
• 1 tablespoon extra•virgin olive oil
• 1 teaspoon Dijon mustard
• 1 teaspoon honey
• 1 clove garlic, minced
• Salt and pepper to taste

Is the recipe easy to follow?

40. Mixed Green Salad with Balsamic Vinaigrette

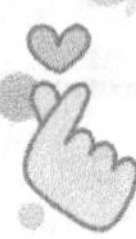

Procedure:

1. In a large salad bowl, combine the mixed greens, cherry tomatoes, cucumber, red onion, feta cheese and toasted almonds.

2. In a small bowl, whisk together the balsamic vinegar, olive oil, Dijon mustard, honey, garlic, salt and pepper to make the vinaigrette.

3. Drizzle the balsamic vinaigrette over the salad and toss gently to coat.

Nutritional Information (per serving):
Calories: 150
Total Carbs: 12g
Fiber: 4g
Net Carbs: 8g
Protein: 6g
Fat: 10g

This salad is packed with nutrient•dense greens, healthy fats from the olive oil and almonds, and a touch of sweetness from the balsamic vinegar and honey. The portion size and nutrient profile make it an excellent choice for a diabetic•friendly meal for seniors. Enjoy!

What is the total cooking time, including prep time?

Prep Time : _______________

Cook Time : _______________

Servings : _______________

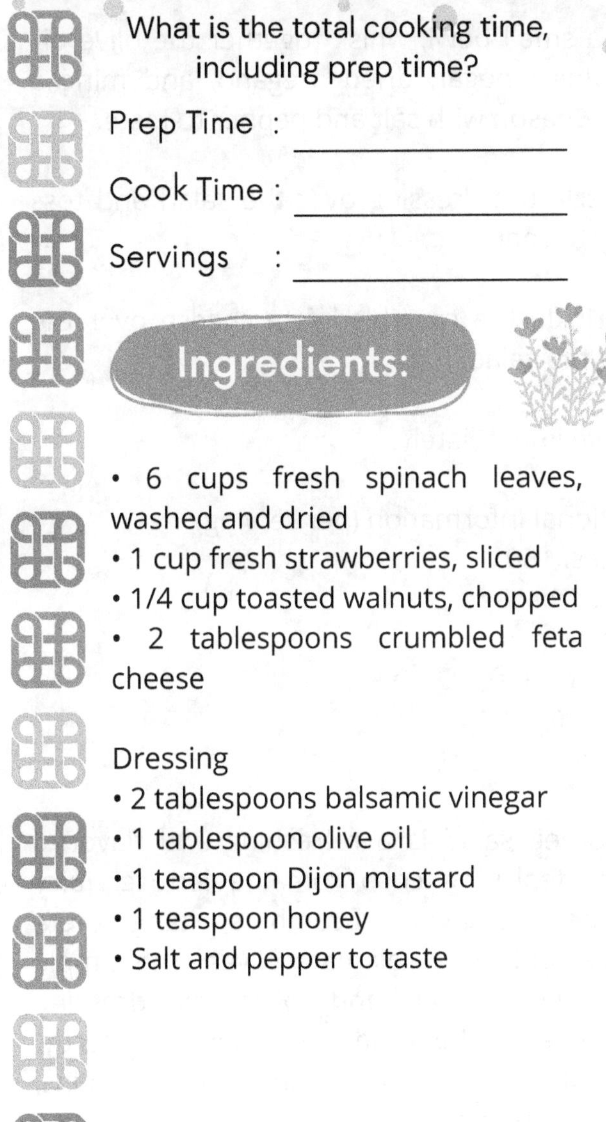

Ingredients:

• 6 cups fresh spinach leaves, washed and dried
• 1 cup fresh strawberries, sliced
• 1/4 cup toasted walnuts, chopped
• 2 tablespoons crumbled feta cheese

Dressing
• 2 tablespoons balsamic vinegar
• 1 tablespoon olive oil
• 1 teaspoon Dijon mustard
• 1 teaspoon honey
• Salt and pepper to taste

Is the recipe easy to follow?

41. Spinach Salad with Strawberries and Walnuts

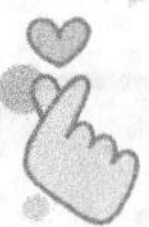

Procedure:

1. In a large salad bowl, combine the spinach leaves, sliced strawberries, chopped walnuts, and crumbled feta cheese.

2. In a small bowl, whisk together the balsamic vinegar, olive oil, Dijon mustard, and honey. Season with salt and pepper to taste.

3. Drizzle the dressing over the salad and toss gently to coat.

4. Serve immediately.

Nutritional Information (per serving):
Calories: 150
Total Carbs: 12g
Fiber: 3g
Net Carbs: 9g
Protein: 5g
Fat: 10g

This spinach salad is a delicious and nutritious option, featuring fresh strawberries, crunchy walnuts, and a tangy balsamic vinaigrette. The combination of the nutrient•dense spinach, heart•healthy walnuts, and antioxidant•rich strawberries makes this a great choice for a light and refreshing meal or side dish.

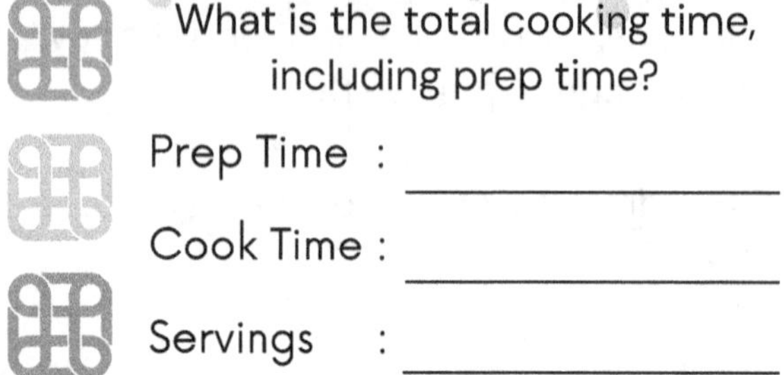

What is the total cooking time, including prep time?

Prep Time : _______________

Cook Time : _______________

Servings : _______________

Ingredients:

• 6 cups chopped romaine lettuce
• 1 cup cherry tomatoes, halved
• 1/2 cup diced cucumber
• 1/4 cup sliced red onion
• 1/4 cup pitted kalamata olives, halved
• 1/4 cup crumbled feta cheese

Dressing
• 2 tablespoons olive oil
• 1 tablespoon red wine vinegar
• 1 teaspoon dried oregano
• 1 clove garlic, minced
• Salt and pepper to taste

Is the recipe easy to follow?

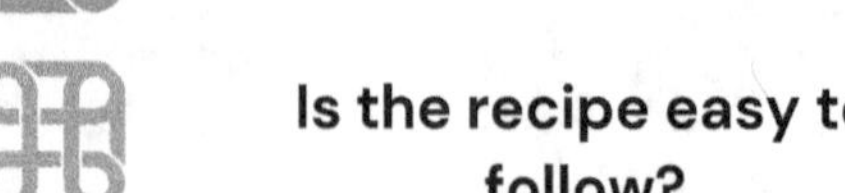
42. Greek Salad with Feta Cheese and Olives

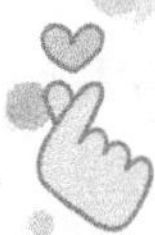

Procedure:

1. In a large salad bowl, combine the chopped romaine lettuce, cherry tomatoes, diced cucumber, sliced red onion, and halved kalamata olives.

2. In a small bowl, whisk together the olive oil, red wine vinegar, dried oregano, and minced garlic. Season with salt and pepper to taste.

3. Drizzle the dressing over the salad and toss gently to coat.

4. Sprinkle the crumbled feta cheese over the top of the salad.

5. Serve immediately.

Nutritional Information (per serving):
Calories: 160
Total Carbs: 8g
Fiber: 2g
Net Carbs: 6g
Protein: 6g
Fat: 13g

This Greek salad is a refreshing and flavorful option, featuring crisp romaine lettuce, juicy tomatoes, crunchy cucumbers, tangy feta cheese, and briny kalamata olives. The simple red wine vinegar and olive oil dressing complements the other ingredients perfectly. This salad is a great source of vitamins, minerals, and healthy fats.

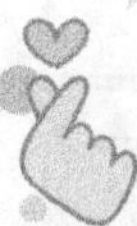

What are the critical points in the recipe (e.g., temperature control, timing)?

What is the total cooking time, including prep time?

Prep Time : _______________

Cook Time : _______________

Servings   : _______________

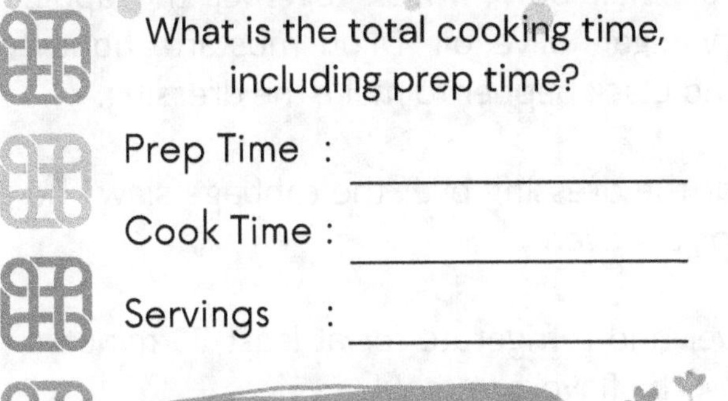

Ingredients:

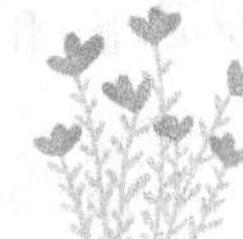

- 6 cups chopped kale, stems removed
- 1 medium apple, cored and diced
- 1/2 cup toasted pecans, chopped
- 2 tablespoons dried cranberries
- 2 tablespoons shredded parmesan cheese

Dressing
- 2 tablespoons olive oil
- 1 tablespoon apple cider vinegar
- 1 teaspoon Dijon mustard
- 1 teaspoon honey
- 1/4 teaspoon salt
- 1/4 teaspoon black pepper

Is the recipe easy to follow?

43. *Kale Salad with Apples and Pecans*

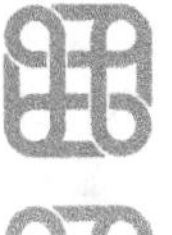

1. In a large salad bowl, combine the chopped kale, diced apple, toasted pecans, dried cranberries, and shredded parmesan cheese.

2. In a small bowl, whisk together the olive oil, apple cider vinegar, Dijon mustard, honey, salt, and black pepper to make the dressing.

3. Pour the dressing over the kale salad and toss to coat evenly.

4. Let the salad sit for 5•10 minutes to allow the kale to soften slightly.

5. Serve immediately.

Nutritional Information (per serving):
Calories: 180
Total Carbs: 15g
Fiber: 3g
Net Carbs: 12g
Protein: 5g
Fat: 13g

This kale salad is a nutrient•dense and flavorful option, featuring the superfood kale, crisp apples, crunchy pecans, and a tangy•sweet dressing. The combination of textures and flavors makes this salad both satisfying and delicious. Kale is packed with vitamins, minerals, and antioxidants, while the apples and pecans provide additional fiber and healthy fats. This salad is a great choice for a light meal or side dish.

What are the critical points in the recipe (e.g., temperature control, timing)?

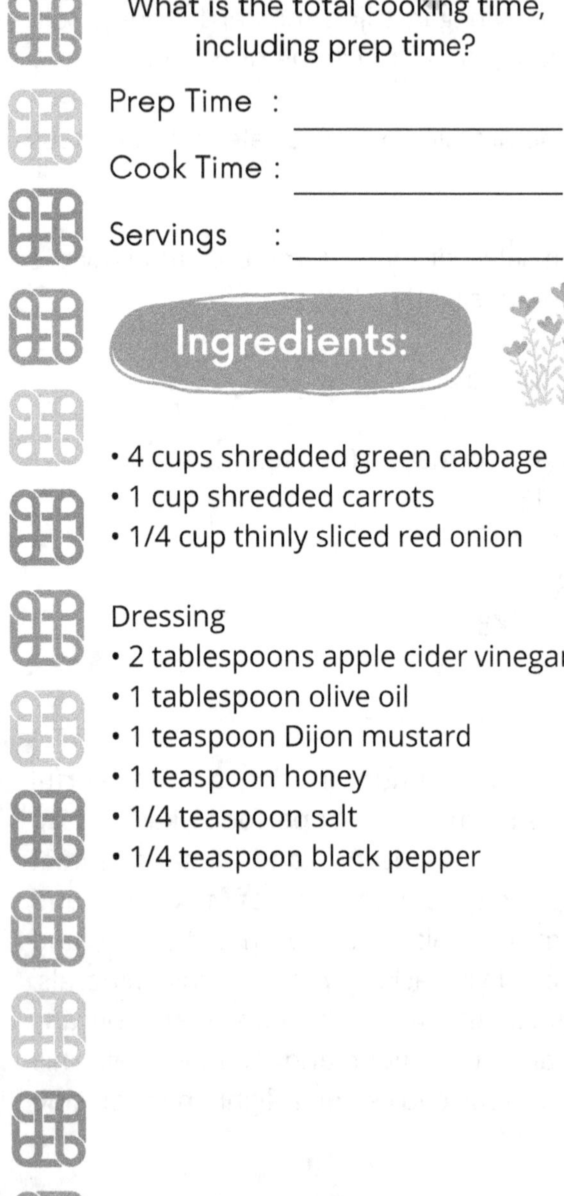

What is the total cooking time, including prep time?

Prep Time : _______________

Cook Time : _______________

Servings   : _______________

Ingredients:

- 4 cups shredded green cabbage
- 1 cup shredded carrots
- 1/4 cup thinly sliced red onion

Dressing
- 2 tablespoons apple cider vinegar
- 1 tablespoon olive oil
- 1 teaspoon Dijon mustard
- 1 teaspoon honey
- 1/4 teaspoon salt
- 1/4 teaspoon black pepper

Is the recipe easy to follow?

44. Cabbage Slaw with Carrots and Apple Cider Vinegar Dressing

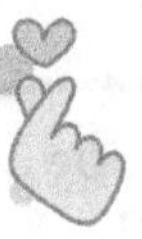

Procedure:

1. In a large bowl, combine the shredded green cabbage, shredded carrots, and thinly sliced red onion.

2. In a small bowl, whisk together the apple cider vinegar, olive oil, Dijon mustard, honey, salt, and black pepper to make the dressing.

3. Pour the dressing over the cabbage slaw and toss to coat evenly.

4. Cover and refrigerate for at least 30 minutes to allow the flavors to meld.

5. Serve chilled or at room temperature.

Nutritional Information (per serving):
Calories: 80
Total Carbs: 10g
Fiber: 3g
Net Carbs: 7g
Protein: 1g
Fat: 4g

This cabbage slaw is a refreshing and crunchy side dish that's perfect for summer. The apple cider vinegar dressing adds a tangy and slightly sweet flavor that complements the fresh vegetables. The carrots and cabbage provide a good source of fiber, vitamins, and antioxidants. This slaw is a great accompaniment to grilled meats, burgers, or as a topping for tacos.

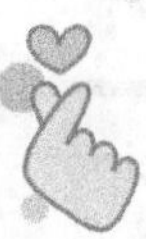

What is the total cooking time, including prep time?

Prep Time : ________________

Cook Time : ________________

Servings   : ________________

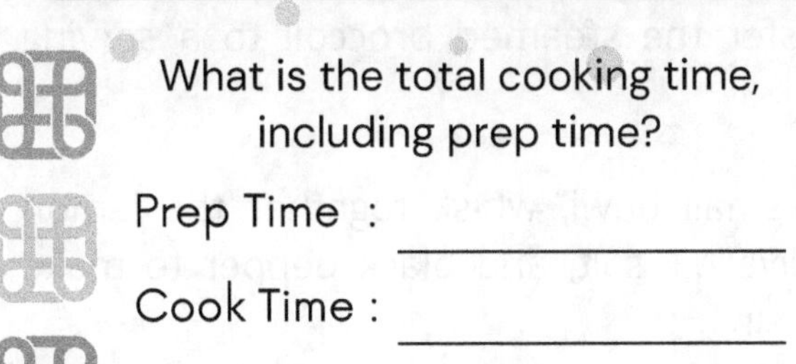

- 5 cups baby arugula
- 1/4 cup shaved Parmesan cheese
- 2 tablespoons toasted pine nuts (optional)

Dressing
- 2 tablespoons fresh lemon juice
- 1 tablespoon extra•virgin olive oil
- 1 teaspoon Dijon mustard
- 1/4 teaspoon salt
- 1/8 teaspoon black pepper

Is the recipe easy to follow?

45. Arugula Salad with Lemon and Parmesan

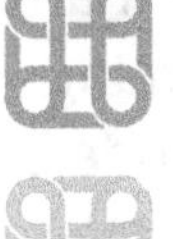
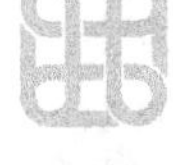
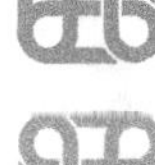
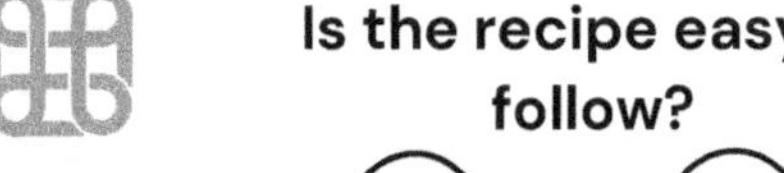

1. In a large salad bowl, combine the baby arugula, shaved Parmesan cheese, and toasted pine nuts (if using).

2. In a small bowl, whisk together the lemon juice, olive oil, Dijon mustard, salt, and black pepper to make the dressing.

3. Drizzle the dressing over the arugula salad and toss gently to coat.

4. Serve immediately.

Nutritional Information (per serving):
Calories: 90
Total Carbs: 3g
Fiber: 1g
Net Carbs: 2g
Protein: 4g
Fat: 7g

This arugula salad is a simple yet flavorful dish that showcases the peppery taste of the arugula. The lemon dressing provides a bright, tangy contrast, while the Parmesan cheese adds a savory, umami element. The optional pine nuts provide a nice crunch. This salad is a great source of vitamins, minerals, and antioxidants, making it a healthy and refreshing choice. Serve it as a side dish or a light main course.

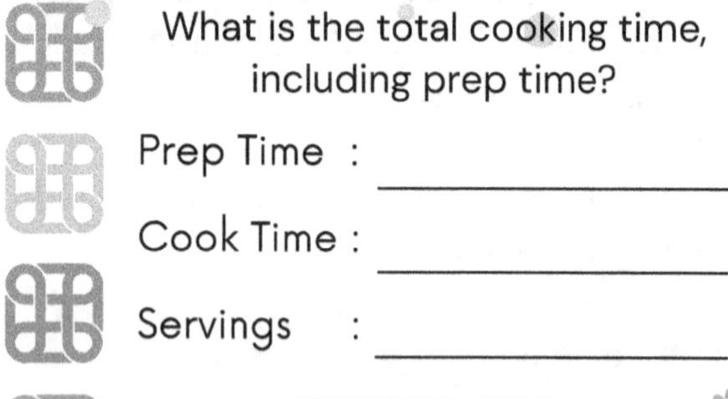

What are the critical points in the recipe (e.g., temperature control, timing)?

What is the total cooking time, including prep time?

Prep Time : _______________

Cook Time : _______________

Servings : _______________

Ingredients:

• 1 lb broccoli florets
• 2 tablespoons water
• 1 tablespoon fresh lemon juice
• 1 teaspoon olive oil
• 1/4 teaspoon salt
• 1/8 teaspoon black pepper

Is the recipe easy to follow?

46. Steamed Broccoli with Lemon

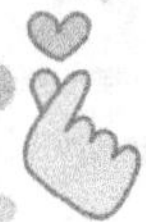

Procedure:

1. In a steamer basket set over a saucepan of simmering water, steam the broccoli florets for 5•7 minutes, or until tender•crisp.

2. Transfer the steamed broccoli to a serving bowl.

3. In a small bowl, whisk together the lemon juice, olive oil, salt, and black pepper to make the dressing.

4. Drizzle the lemon dressing over the steamed broccoli and toss gently to coat.

5. Serve the broccoli warm or at room temperature.

Nutritional Information (per serving):
Calories: 60
Total Carbs: 6g
Fiber: 3g
Net Carbs: 3g
Protein: 3g
Fat: 3g

This simple steamed broccoli dish is a great way to enjoy the natural flavors of the vegetable. The lemon dressing adds a bright, tangy note that complements the broccoli perfectly. Steaming helps to preserve the nutrients and crisp•tender texture of the broccoli. This side dish is low in calories and carbs, making it a healthy option to serve alongside a variety of main dishes.

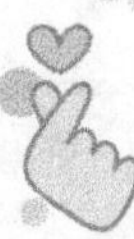

What are the critical points in the recipe (e.g., temperature control, timing)?

What is the total cooking time, including prep time?

Prep Time : _______________

Cook Time : _______________

Servings   : _______________

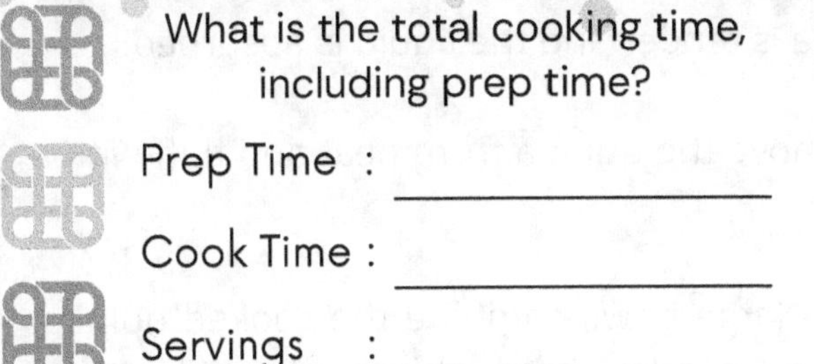

Ingredients:

• 1 lb Brussels sprouts, trimmed and halved
• 2 tablespoons olive oil
• 1/2 teaspoon salt
• 1/4 teaspoon black pepper

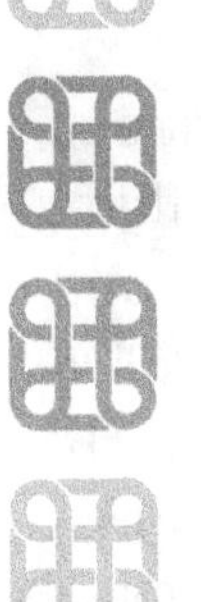

Is the recipe easy to follow?

47. Roasted Brussels Sprouts with Olive Oil

1. Preheat your oven to 400°F (200°C).

2. In a large bowl, toss the trimmed and halved Brussels sprouts with the olive oil, salt, and black pepper until the sprouts are evenly coated.

3. Spread the Brussels sprouts in a single layer on a large baking sheet lined with parchment paper or a silicone baking mat.

4. Roast the Brussels sprouts in the preheated oven for 20·25 minutes, tossing halfway through, until they are tender and lightly browned.

5. Serve the roasted Brussels sprouts hot, as a side dish.

Nutritional Information (per serving):
Calories: 80
Total Carbs: 7g
Fiber: 3g
Net Carbs: 4g
Protein: 3g
Fat: 5g

These roasted Brussels sprouts are a simple and delicious way to enjoy this nutritious vegetable. The olive oil helps to crisp up the outer leaves while keeping the insides tender. The salt and pepper provide a basic seasoning, but you can also experiment with other herbs and spices to customize the flavor. Roasting brings out the natural sweetness of the Brussels sprouts, making them a great side dish for a variety of meals.

What are the critical points in the recipe (e.g., temperature control, timing)?

What is the total cooking time, including prep time?

Prep Time : ___________________

Cook Time : ___________________

Servings   : ___________________

Ingredients:

• 1 cup uncooked quinoa, rinsed
• 2 cups vegetable or chicken broth
• 1/4 cup chopped fresh parsley
• 2 tablespoons chopped fresh basil
• 2 tablespoons chopped fresh chives
• 1 tablespoon olive oil
• 1 tablespoon lemon juice
• 1/2 teaspoon salt
• 1/4 teaspoon black pepper

Is the recipe easy to follow?

☺   ☹

48. Quinoa with Fresh Herbs

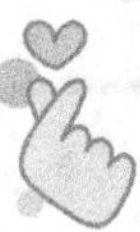

1. In a medium saucepan, combine the rinsed quinoa and broth. Bring to a boil over high heat.

2. Once boiling, reduce the heat to low, cover, and simmer for 15•20 minutes, or until the quinoa is tender and the liquid is absorbed.

3. Remove the quinoa from heat and fluff with a fork.

4. In a large bowl, combine the cooked quinoa, chopped parsley, basil, chives, olive oil, lemon juice, salt, and black pepper. Toss gently to mix.

5. Serve the quinoa with fresh herbs warm or at room temperature.

Nutritional Information (per serving):
Calories: 180
Total Carbs: 26g
Fiber: 3g
Net Carbs: 23g
Protein: 6g
Fat: 6g

This quinoa dish is a delicious and nutritious side or main course. The combination of fluffy quinoa and fresh herbs like parsley, basil, and chives creates a bright, flavorful dish. The olive oil and lemon juice add a light, refreshing touch. Quinoa is a complete protein and a good source of fiber, making this a wholesome and satisfying option. Serve it alongside grilled meats, roasted vegetables, or enjoy it on its own.

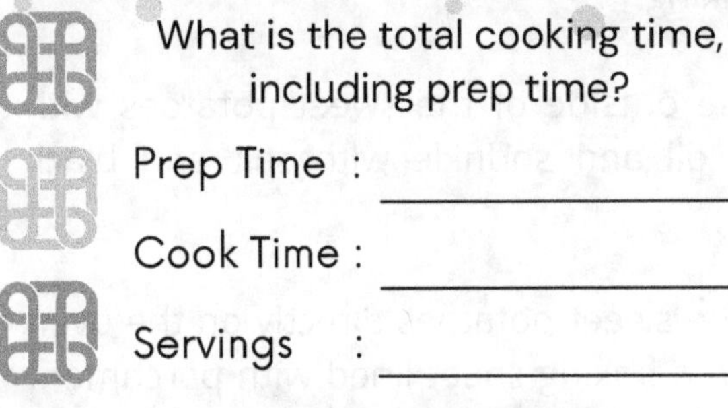

What is the total cooking time, including prep time?

Prep Time : ___________________

Cook Time : ___________________

Servings : ___________________

Ingredients:

• 1 large head of cauliflower, cut into florets (about 6 cups)
• 2 tablespoons unsalted butter
• 2 tablespoons full•fat cream cheese
• 1/4 cup unsweetened almond milk (or regular milk)
• 1/2 teaspoon garlic powder
• 1/4 teaspoon salt
• 1/8 teaspoon black pepper

Is the recipe easy to follow?

49. Mashed Cauliflower

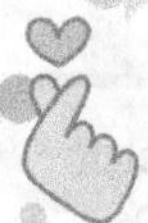

Procedure:

1. In a large pot, bring 1 inch of water to a boil. Add the cauliflower florets, cover, and steam for 10•12 minutes, until very tender.

2. Drain the cauliflower and transfer it to a food processor or high•powered blender.

3. Add the butter, cream cheese, almond milk, garlic powder, salt, and black pepper to the food processor.

4. Blend or process the cauliflower mixture until smooth and creamy, scraping down the sides as needed.

5. Taste and adjust seasoning as desired.

6. Serve the mashed cauliflower warm.

Nutritional Information (per serving):
Calories: 100
Total Carbs: 7g
Fiber: 3g
Net Carbs: 4g
Protein: 3g
Fat: 7g

This mashed cauliflower is a delicious and low•carb alternative to traditional mashed potatoes. The cauliflower provides a creamy texture, while the butter, cream cheese, and almond milk add richness and creaminess. The garlic powder, salt, and pepper provide simple seasoning. Mashed cauliflower is a great side dish that can be enjoyed by those following a keto or low•carb diet.

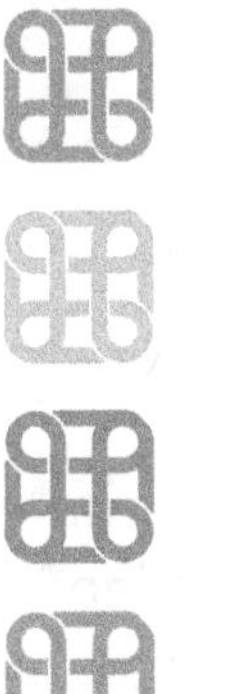

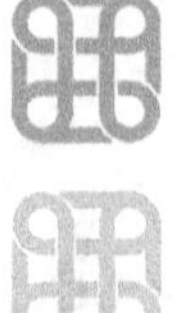
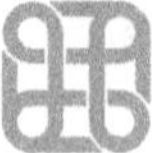

What is the total cooking time, including prep time?

Prep Time : _______________

Cook Time : _______________

Servings : _______________

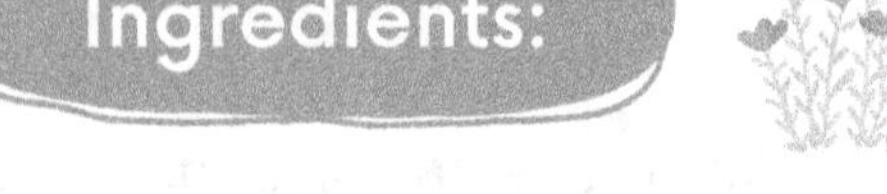

Ingredients:

- 4 medium sweet potatoes, scrubbed clean
- 1 tablespoon olive oil
- 1/2 teaspoon salt
- 1/4 teaspoon black pepper

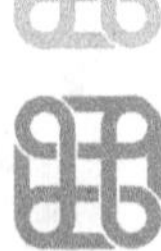
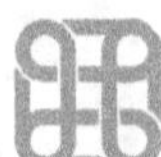
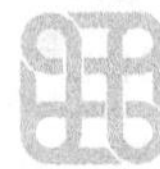
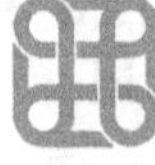
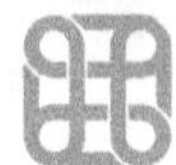
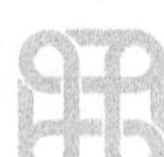

Is the recipe easy to follow?

50. Baked Sweet Potato

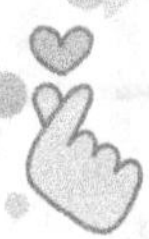

Procedure:

1. Preheat your oven to 400°F (200°C).

2. Use a fork to poke several holes all over the sweet potatoes. This will allow steam to escape during baking.

3. Rub the outside of the sweet potatoes with the olive oil and sprinkle with salt and black pepper.

4. Place the sweet potatoes directly on the oven rack or on a baking sheet lined with parchment paper.

5. Bake for 45•60 minutes, or until a knife can easily pierce through the center. The sweet potatoes should be very soft when squeezed.

6. Remove the baked sweet potatoes from the oven and let them cool for 5 minutes.

7. Slice open the sweet potatoes and serve warm, with desired toppings (such as butter, cinnamon, or a drizzle of honey).

Nutritional Information (per serving):
Calories: 150
Total Carbs: 27g
Fiber: 4g
Net Carbs: 23g
Protein: 3g
Fat: 3g

Baked sweet potatoes are a simple and nutritious side dish. They are an excellent source of vitamins A and C, as well as fiber and complex carbohydrates. The natural sweetness of the sweet potato pairs well with savory or sweet toppings. This basic baked sweet potato recipe is easy to prepare and can be customized to your liking.

What is the total cooking time, including prep time?

Prep Time : _______________

Cook Time : _______________

Servings   : _______________

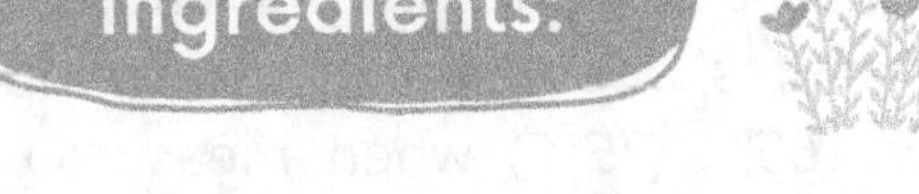

Ingredients:

- 1 lb fresh green beans, trimmed
- 1 tablespoon olive oil
- 1/4 cup sliced almonds
- 2 cloves garlic, minced
- 1/4 teaspoon salt
- 1/8 teaspoon black pepper

Is the recipe easy to follow?

51. Green Beans with Almonds

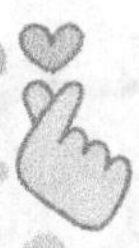

Procedure:

1. Bring a large pot of salted water to a boil. Add the trimmed green beans and cook for 5•7 minutes, until tender•crisp. Drain the beans and set aside.

2. In a large skillet, heat the olive oil over medium heat. Add the sliced almonds and cook for 2•3 minutes, stirring frequently, until lightly toasted.

3. Add the minced garlic to the skillet and cook for 1 minute, until fragrant.

4. Add the cooked green beans to the skillet and toss to combine. Season with salt and black pepper.

5. Cook for an additional 2•3 minutes, stirring occasionally, until the beans are heated through.

6. Serve the green beans with almonds warm.

Nutritional Information (per serving):
Calories: 90
Total Carbs: 7g
Fiber: 3g
Net Carbs: 4g
Protein: 3g
Fat: 6g

This simple green bean dish is a delicious and nutritious side. The crunchy almonds and garlic add great flavor and texture to the tender•crisp green beans. The olive oil provides healthy fats, while the beans are a good source of fiber, vitamins, and minerals. This recipe is easy to prepare and pairs well with a variety of main dishes.

What are the critical points in the recipe (e.g., temperature control, timing)?

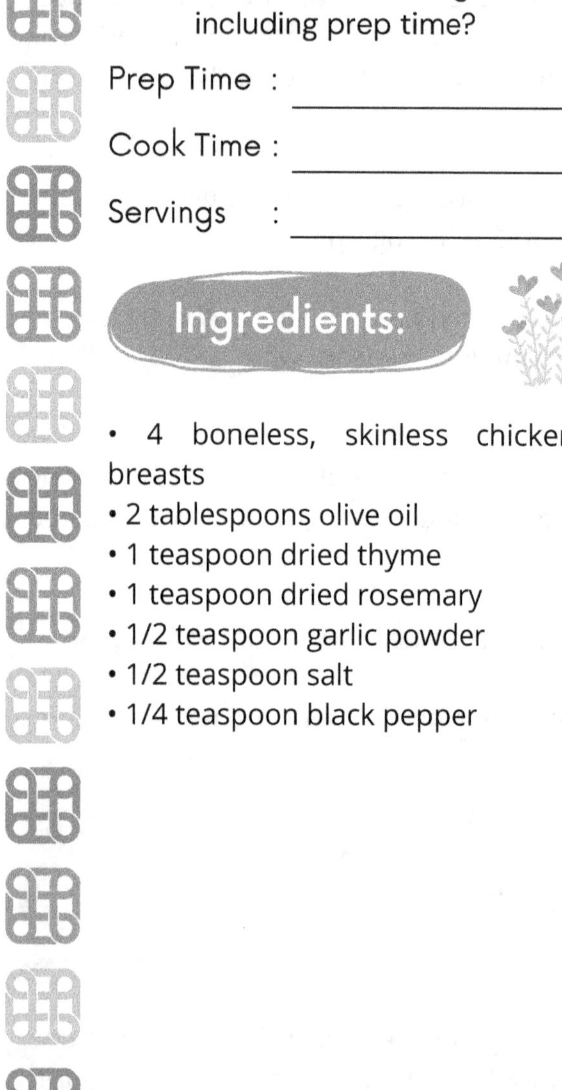

What is the total cooking time, including prep time?

Prep Time : _______________

Cook Time : _______________

Servings   : _______________

Ingredients:

- 4 boneless, skinless chicken breasts
- 2 tablespoons olive oil
- 1 teaspoon dried thyme
- 1 teaspoon dried rosemary
- 1/2 teaspoon garlic powder
- 1/2 teaspoon salt
- 1/4 teaspoon black pepper

Is the recipe easy to follow?

52. Baked Chicken Breast with Herbs

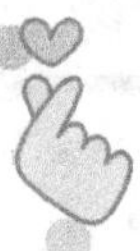

Procedure:

1. Preheat your oven to 400°F (200°C).

2. Pat the chicken breasts dry with paper towels and place them in a baking dish or on a rimmed baking sheet.

3. In a small bowl, mix together the olive oil, dried thyme, dried rosemary, garlic powder, salt, and black pepper.

4. Brush or rub the herb mixture evenly over the top and sides of the chicken breasts.

5. Bake the chicken in the preheated oven for 25•30 minutes, or until the internal temperature reaches 165°F (75°C) when measured with a meat thermometer.

6. Remove the baked chicken from the oven and let it rest for 5 minutes before serving.

Nutritional Information (per serving):
Calories: 200
Total Carbs: 0g
Fiber: 0g
Net Carbs: 0g
Protein: 30g
Fat: 8g

This baked chicken breast with herbs is a simple and flavorful dish that's easy to prepare. The combination of thyme, rosemary, and garlic creates a delicious seasoning that complements the lean chicken perfectly. Baking the chicken ensures it stays moist and juicy. Serve this dish with roasted vegetables or a fresh salad for a complete and healthy meal.

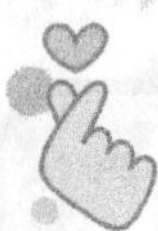

What are the critical points in the recipe (e.g., temperature control, timing)?

What is the total cooking time, including prep time?

Prep Time : _______________

Cook Time : _______________

Servings   : _______________

Ingredients:

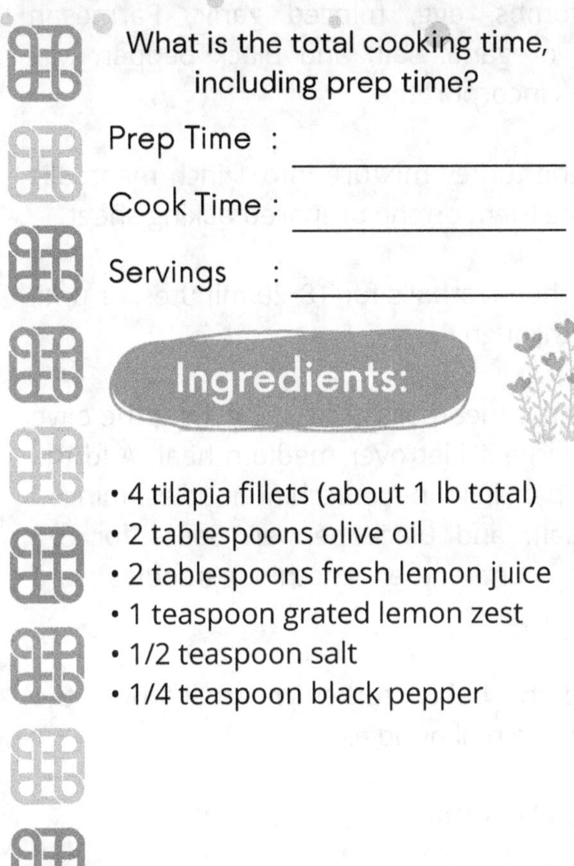

- 4 tilapia fillets (about 1 lb total)
- 2 tablespoons olive oil
- 2 tablespoons fresh lemon juice
- 1 teaspoon grated lemon zest
- 1/2 teaspoon salt
- 1/4 teaspoon black pepper

Is the recipe easy to follow?

53. Grilled Tilapia with Lemon

1. Preheat your grill or grill pan to medium·high heat.

2. In a shallow dish, combine the olive oil, lemon juice, lemon zest, salt, and black pepper. Add the tilapia fillets and turn to coat both sides with the marinade.

3. Grill the tilapia for 3·4 minutes per side, or until the fish flakes easily with a fork and is opaque throughout.

4. Transfer the grilled tilapia fillets to a serving plate.

5. Serve the grilled tilapia warm, with any remaining lemon marinade drizzled over the top.

Nutritional Information (per serving):
Calories: 180
Total Carbs: 0g
Fiber: 0g
Net Carbs: 0g
Protein: 30g
Fat: 8g

This grilled tilapia with lemon is a simple and delicious way to prepare this lean, mild·flavored fish. The lemon marinade adds a bright, tangy flavor that complements the tilapia perfectly. Tilapia is a great source of protein and is low in calories and carbs, making it a healthy choice. Grilling the fish gives it a nice, flaky texture. Serve this dish with a side of roasted vegetables or a fresh salad for a complete and nutritious meal.

What is the total cooking time, including prep time?

Prep Time : _______________

Cook Time : _______________

Servings   : _______________

Ingredients:

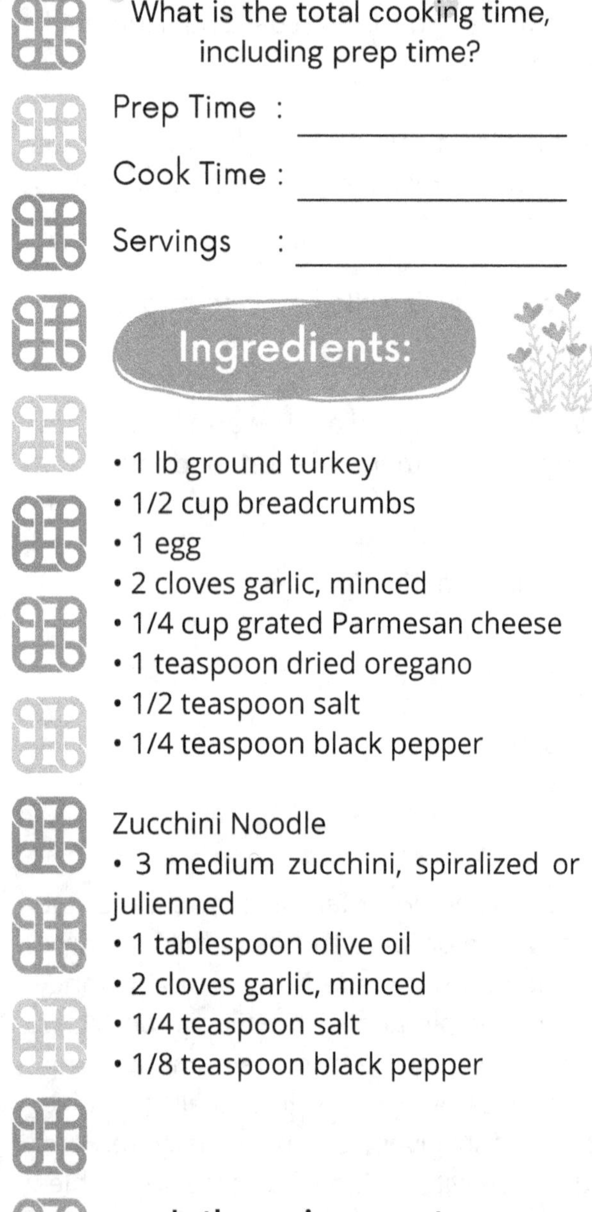

- 1 lb ground turkey
- 1/2 cup breadcrumbs
- 1 egg
- 2 cloves garlic, minced
- 1/4 cup grated Parmesan cheese
- 1 teaspoon dried oregano
- 1/2 teaspoon salt
- 1/4 teaspoon black pepper

Zucchini Noodle
- 3 medium zucchini, spiralized or julienned
- 1 tablespoon olive oil
- 2 cloves garlic, minced
- 1/4 teaspoon salt
- 1/8 teaspoon black pepper

Is the recipe easy to follow?

54. *Turkey Meatballs with Zucchini Noodles*

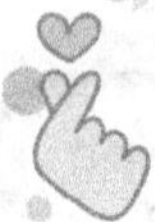

Procedure:

1. Preheat your oven to 400°F (200°C). Line a baking sheet with parchment paper.

2. In a large bowl, combine the ground turkey, breadcrumbs, egg, minced garlic, Parmesan cheese, oregano, salt, and black pepper. Mix until well incorporated.

3. Roll the turkey mixture into 1•inch meatballs and place them on the prepared baking sheet.

4. Bake the meatballs for 18•20 minutes, or until cooked through.

5. While the meatballs are baking, heat the olive oil in a large skillet over medium heat. Add the spiralized or julienned zucchini noodles, minced garlic, salt, and black pepper. Sauté for 3•5 minutes, until the zucchini noodles are tender•crisp.

6. Serve the baked turkey meatballs over the sautéed zucchini noodles.

Nutritional Information (per serving):
Calories: 250
Total Carbs: 12g
Fiber: 3g
Net Carbs: 9g
Protein: 25g
Fat: 12g

This turkey meatball and zucchini noodle dish is a healthy and delicious low•carb meal. The turkey meatballs are flavorful and tender, while the zucchini noodles provide a nutritious and low•calorie alternative to traditional pasta. This dish is easy to prepare and can be a great option for those following a keto or low•carb diet.

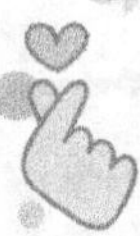

Procedure:

What is the total cooking time, including prep time?

Prep Time : _______________

Cook Time : _______________

Servings   : _______________

Ingredients:

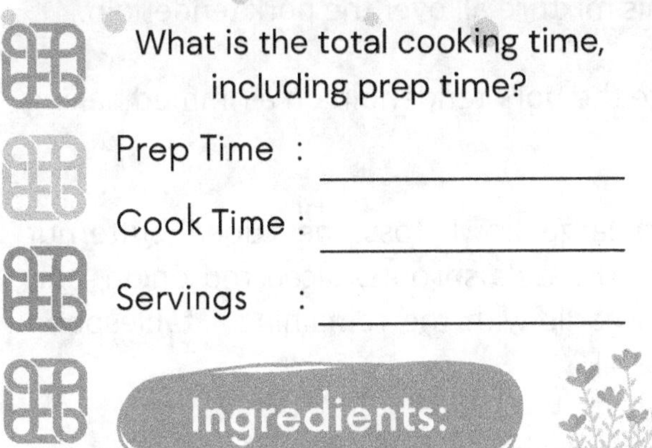

- 1 medium head green cabbage
- 1 lb ground turkey or lean ground beef
- 1 cup cooked brown rice
- 1 egg, beaten
- 1/2 cup diced onion
- 2 cloves garlic, minced
- 1 teaspoon dried oregano
- 1/2 teaspoon salt
- 1/4 teaspoon black pepper
- 1 (15 oz) can tomato sauce
- 1/4 cup water

Is the recipe easy to follow?

55. Stuffed Cabbage Rolls

1. Bring a large pot of water to a boil. Add the whole head of cabbage and cook for 3•5 minutes, until the outer leaves are softened. Remove the cabbage from the water and let it cool slightly.

2. Carefully peel off the softened cabbage leaves, keeping them intact. You should have about 12•14 leaves.

3. In a large bowl, combine the ground turkey/beef, cooked brown rice, beaten egg, diced onion, minced garlic, oregano, salt, and black pepper. Mix well.

4. Place about 2•3 tablespoons of the meat mixture onto the center of each cabbage leaf. Fold the sides of the leaf over the filling and then roll up tightly.

5. Arrange the stuffed cabbage rolls seam•side down in a baking dish.

6. In a small bowl, mix together the tomato sauce and water. Pour the sauce over the stuffed cabbage rolls.

7. Cover the baking dish with foil and bake at 375°F (190°C) for 45•55 minutes, until the cabbage rolls are heated through and the filling is cooked. Serve the stuffed cabbage rolls warm.

These stuffed cabbage rolls are a delicious and healthy meal. The ground turkey or beef filling, combined with brown rice and vegetables, provides a balance of protein, complex carbohydrates, and fiber. The cabbage leaves act as a low•carb wrapper, and the tomato sauce adds a flavorful touch. This dish is easy to prepare and can be a great option for a family dinner or meal prep.

What is the total cooking time, including prep time?

Prep Time : _______________

Cook Time : _______________

Servings : _______________

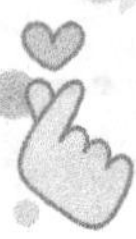

Ingredients:

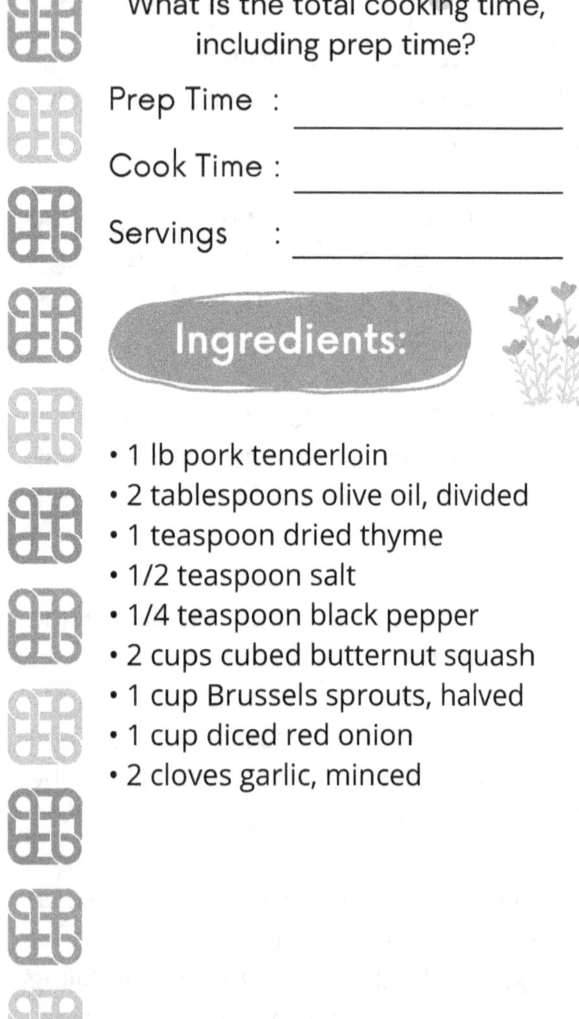

- 1 lb pork tenderloin
- 2 tablespoons olive oil, divided
- 1 teaspoon dried thyme
- 1/2 teaspoon salt
- 1/4 teaspoon black pepper
- 2 cups cubed butternut squash
- 1 cup Brussels sprouts, halved
- 1 cup diced red onion
- 2 cloves garlic, minced

Is the recipe easy to follow?

56. Pork Tenderloin with Roasted Vegetables

Procedure:

1. Preheat your oven to 400°F (200°C).

2. In a small bowl, combine 1 tablespoon of the olive oil, dried thyme, salt, and black pepper. Rub this mixture all over the pork tenderloin.

3. Place the pork tenderloin on a rimmed baking sheet.

4. In a large bowl, toss the cubed butternut squash, Brussels sprouts, diced red onion, and minced garlic with the remaining 1 tablespoon of olive oil.

5. Spread the seasoned vegetables around the pork tenderloin on the baking sheet.

6. Roast the pork and vegetables in the preheated oven for 25•30 minutes, or until the pork reaches an internal temperature of 145°F (63°C).

7. Remove the pork tenderloin from the oven and let it rest for 5 minutes before slicing.

8. Serve the sliced pork tenderloin with the roasted vegetables.

This pork tenderloin with roasted vegetables is a delicious and nutritious meal. The pork is seasoned with thyme, salt, and pepper, while the vegetables (butternut squash, Brussels sprouts, and onion) provide a variety of vitamins, minerals, and fiber. Roasting the vegetables brings out their natural sweetness and creates a flavorful, caramelized texture. This dish is easy to prepare and makes for a well•balanced, low•carb dinner.

What is the total cooking time, including prep time?

Prep Time : _______________

Cook Time : _______________

Servings : _______________

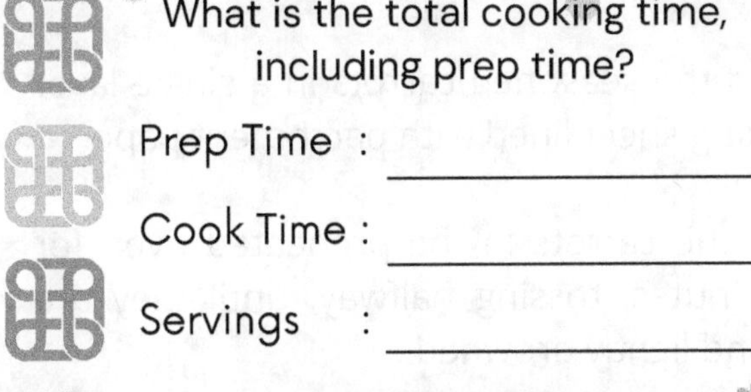

Ingredients:

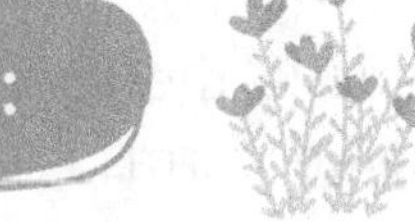

- 8 large eggs
- 1/4 cup unsweetened almond milk
- 1/4 teaspoon salt
- 1/8 teaspoon black pepper
- 1 tablespoon olive oil
- 1 cup diced bell pepper
- 1 cup sliced mushrooms
- 1 cup chopped spinach
- 1/4 cup shredded cheddar cheese

Is the recipe easy to follow?

57. Vegetable Frittata

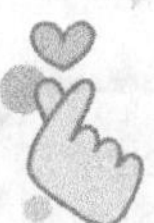

Procedure:

1. Preheat your oven to 375°F (190°C).

2. In a medium bowl, whisk together the eggs, almond milk, salt, and black pepper until well combined.

3. In a 9-inch oven-safe non-stick skillet, heat the olive oil over medium heat. Add the diced bell pepper, sliced mushrooms, and chopped spinach. Sauté for 5-7 minutes, until the vegetables are tender.

4. Pour the egg mixture over the sautéed vegetables in the skillet. Sprinkle the shredded cheddar cheese evenly over the top.

5. Transfer the skillet to the preheated oven and bake for 18-22 minutes, or until the frittata is set and the cheese is melted.

6. Remove the frittata from the oven and let it cool for 5 minutes. Slice and serve the vegetable frittata warm.

Nutritional Information (per serving):
Calories: 180
Total Carbs: 6g
Fiber: 2g
Net Carbs: 4g
Protein: 14g
Fat: 12g

This vegetable frittata is a delicious and nutritious breakfast or brunch option. The combination of eggs, vegetables, and cheese provides a balance of protein, fiber, and healthy fats. The bell pepper, mushrooms, and spinach add a variety of vitamins, minerals, and antioxidants. This frittata is easy to prepare and can be customized with your choice of vegetables.

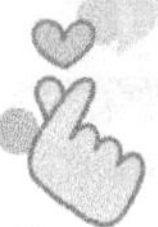

What is the total cooking time, including prep time?

Prep Time : _________________

Cook Time : _________________

Servings   : _________________

Ingredients:

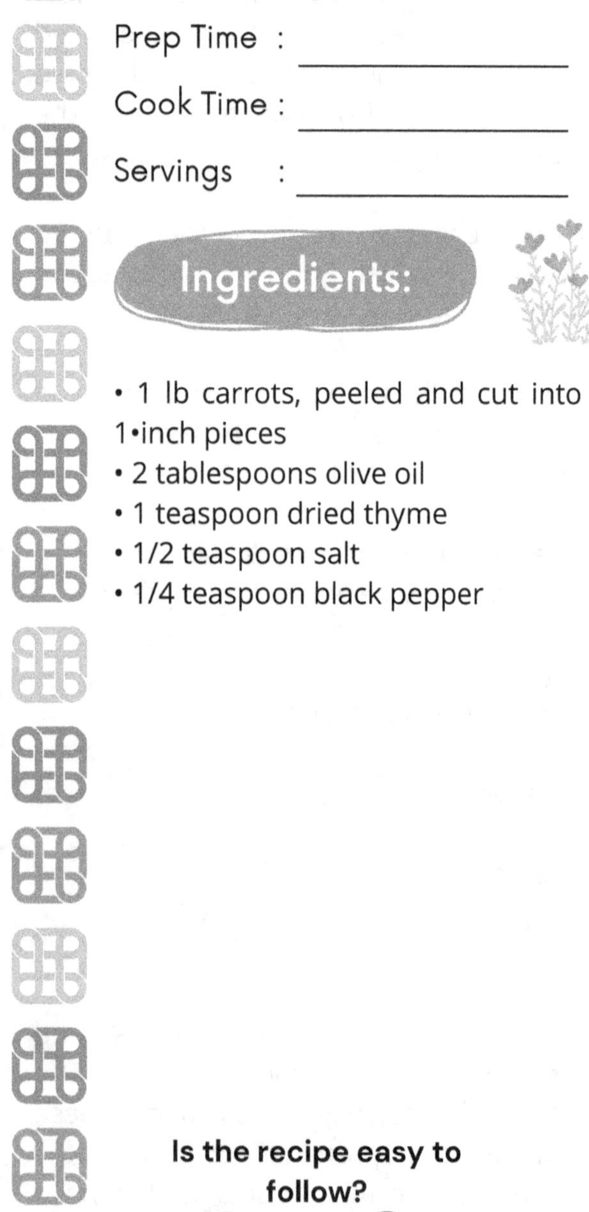

- 1 lb carrots, peeled and cut into 1•inch pieces
- 2 tablespoons olive oil
- 1 teaspoon dried thyme
- 1/2 teaspoon salt
- 1/4 teaspoon black pepper

Is the recipe easy to follow?

58. Roasted Carrots with Thyme

1. Preheat your oven to 400°F (200°C).

2. In a large bowl, toss the peeled and cut carrots with the olive oil, dried thyme, salt, and black pepper until the carrots are evenly coated.

3. Spread the seasoned carrots in a single layer on a baking sheet lined with parchment paper.

4. Roast the carrots in the preheated oven for 20•25 minutes, tossing halfway, until they are tender and lightly browned.

5. Remove the roasted carrots from the oven and serve warm.

Nutritional Information (per serving):
Calories: 100
Total Carbs: 12g
Fiber: 3g
Net Carbs: 9g
Protein: 1g
Fat: 5g

These roasted carrots with thyme are a simple and flavorful side dish. The thyme adds an earthy, aromatic note that complements the natural sweetness of the carrots. Roasting the carrots brings out their natural sugars and creates a delicious, caramelized texture. This dish is easy to prepare and makes a great accompaniment to grilled or roasted meats, fish, or as part of a vegetarian meal. The carrots are a good source of vitamins, minerals, and fiber.

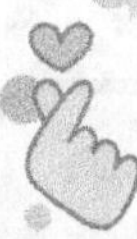

What are the critical points in the recipe (e.g., temperature control, timing)?

What is the total cooking time, including prep time?

Prep Time : _______________

Cook Time : _______________

Servings   : _______________

Ingredients:

- 1 lb fresh spinach, washed and stems removed
- 1 tablespoon olive oil
- 3 cloves garlic, minced
- 1/4 teaspoon salt
- 1/8 teaspoon black pepper

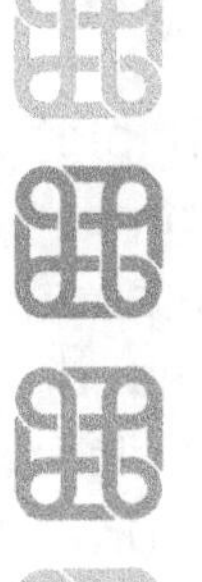
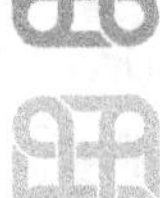
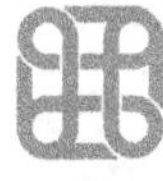
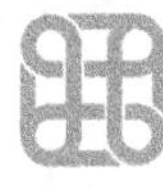

Is the recipe easy to follow?

59. Sautéed Spinach with Garlic

1. In a large skillet or wok, heat the olive oil over medium heat.

2. Add the minced garlic to the hot oil and sauté for 1•2 minutes, until fragrant.

3. Add the fresh spinach to the skillet in batches, if needed, and sauté for 2•3 minutes, stirring frequently, until the spinach is wilted and tender.

4. Season the sautéed spinach with salt and black pepper.

5. Serve the sautéed spinach with garlic warm.

Nutritional Information (per serving):
Calories: 50
Total Carbs: 3g
Fiber: 2g
Net Carbs: 1g
Protein: 3g
Fat: 3g

This sautéed spinach with garlic is a simple and delicious side dish. Spinach is an excellent source of vitamins, minerals, and antioxidants, making it a nutritious addition to any meal. The garlic adds a savory, aromatic flavor that complements the spinach perfectly. This dish comes together quickly and is a great way to incorporate more leafy greens into your diet. Serve it alongside grilled or roasted meats, fish, or as a vegetarian main course.

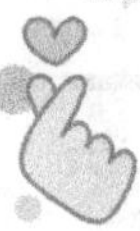

What is the total cooking time,
including prep time?

Prep Time : _______________

Cook Time : _______________

Servings   : _______________

Ingredients:

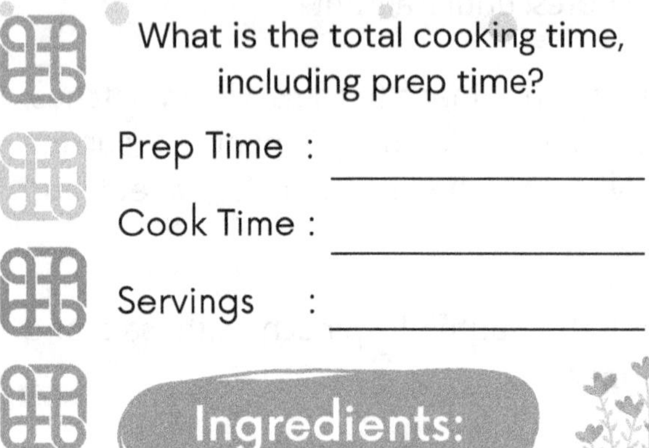

• 2 medium zucchini, sliced lengthwise into 1/2•inch thick strips
• 2 medium yellow squash, sliced lengthwise into 1/2•inch thick strips
• 2 tablespoons olive oil
• 1 teaspoon dried oregano
• 1/2 teaspoon salt
• 1/4 teaspoon black pepper

1. Preheat your grill or grill pan to medium•high heat.

2. In a large bowl, toss the zucchini and yellow squash strips with the olive oil, dried oregano, salt, and black pepper until evenly coated.

3. Grill the zucchini and squash slices for 3•4 minutes per side, or until they are tender and have grill marks.

4. Transfer the grilled zucchini and squash to a serving platter.

5. Serve the grilled vegetables warm.

Nutritional Information (per serving):
Calories: 80
Total Carbs: 6g
Fiber: 2g
Net Carbs: 4g
Protein: 2g
Fat: 6g

This grilled zucchini and squash dish is a simple and delicious way to enjoy these summer vegetables. The combination of zucchini and yellow squash provides a variety of colors and flavors. Grilling the vegetables adds a nice smoky char and brings out their natural sweetness. The oregano, salt, and pepper provide a simple seasoning that complements the vegetables perfectly. This dish is a great low•carb, keto•friendly side or can be served as a light main course.

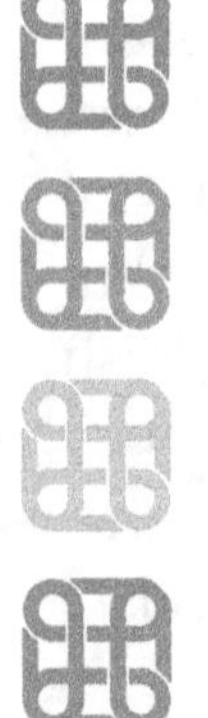

Is the recipe easy to follow?

60. Grilled Zucchini and Squash

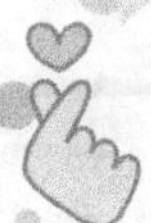

What is the total cooking time,
including prep time?

Prep Time : ________________

Cook Time : ________________

Servings   : ________________

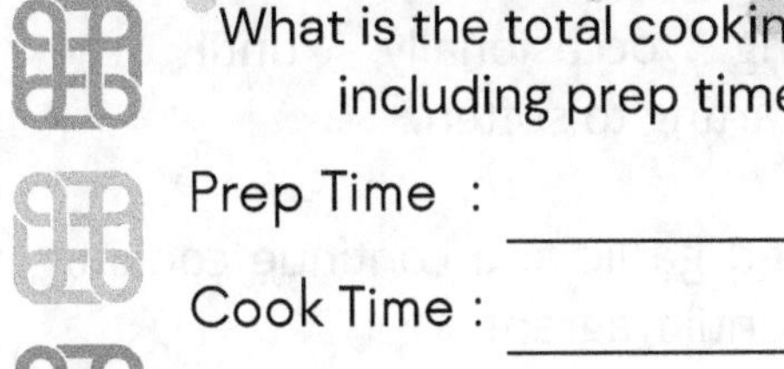

Ingredients:

• 1 large head of cauliflower, cut into florets (about 6 cups)
• 2 tablespoons unsalted butter
• 2 tablespoons full•fat cream cheese
• 1/4 cup unsweetened almond milk (or regular milk)
• 1/2 teaspoon garlic powder
• 1/4 teaspoon salt
• 1/8 teaspoon black pepper

1. In a large pot, bring 1 inch of water to a boil. Add the cauliflower florets, cover, and steam for 10•12 minutes, until very tender.

2. Drain the cauliflower and transfer it to a food processor or high•powered blender.

3. Add the butter, cream cheese, almond milk, garlic powder, salt, and black pepper to the food processor.

4. Blend or process the cauliflower mixture until smooth and creamy, scraping down the sides as needed.

5. Taste and adjust seasoning as desired.

6. Serve the cauliflower mash warm.

Nutritional Information (per serving):
Calories: 100
Total Carbs: 6g
Fiber: 3g
Net Carbs: 3g
Protein: 3g
Fat: 7g

This cauliflower mash is a delicious and low•carb alternative to traditional mashed potatoes. The cauliflower provides a creamy texture, while the butter, cream cheese, and almond milk add richness and creaminess. The garlic powder, salt, and pepper provide simple seasoning. Cauliflower mash is a great side dish that can be enjoyed by those following a keto or low•carb diet.

Is the recipe easy to follow?

61. Cauliflower Mash

What are the critical points in the recipe (e.g., temperature control, timing)?

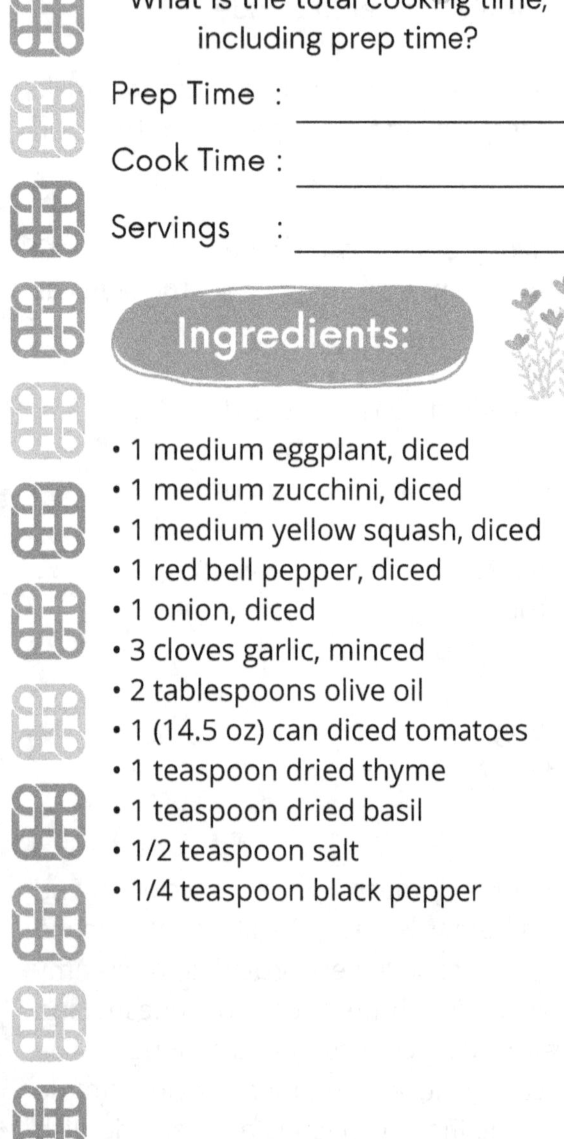

What is the total cooking time, including prep time?

Prep Time : _______________

Cook Time : _______________

Servings : _______________

Ingredients:

- 1 medium eggplant, diced
- 1 medium zucchini, diced
- 1 medium yellow squash, diced
- 1 red bell pepper, diced
- 1 onion, diced
- 3 cloves garlic, minced
- 2 tablespoons olive oil
- 1 (14.5 oz) can diced tomatoes
- 1 teaspoon dried thyme
- 1 teaspoon dried basil
- 1/2 teaspoon salt
- 1/4 teaspoon black pepper

Is the recipe easy to follow?

62. Ratatouille

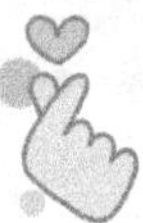

Procedure:

1. In a large skillet or Dutch oven, heat the olive oil over medium heat.

2. Add the diced eggplant, zucchini, yellow squash, bell pepper, and onion. Sauté for 8•10 minutes, stirring occasionally, until the vegetables are starting to soften.

3. Add the minced garlic and continue cooking for 1•2 minutes, until fragrant.

4. Pour in the can of diced tomatoes, including the juices. Stir in the dried thyme, dried basil, salt, and black pepper.

5. Reduce the heat to low, cover the skillet, and simmer for 20•25 minutes, stirring occasionally, until the vegetables are very tender.

6. Serve the ratatouille warm, as a side dish or main course.

Nutritional Information (per serving):
Calories: 120
Total Carbs: 14g
Fiber: 5g
Net Carbs: 9g
Protein: 3g
Fat: 7g

Ratatouille is a classic French vegetable stew that is packed with flavor and nutrients. The combination of eggplant, zucchini, squash, bell pepper, and tomatoes creates a delicious and colorful dish. The herbs and garlic add depth of flavor, while the long simmering time allows the vegetables to become tender and the flavors to meld together. Ratatouille is a great option for a vegetarian or vegan main course, or it can be served as a flavorful side dish.

What are the critical points in the recipe (e.g., temperature control, timing)?

What is the total cooking time, including prep time?

Prep Time : ________________

Cook Time : ________________

Servings   : ________________

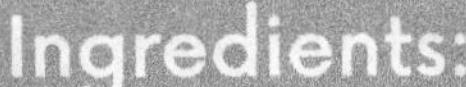 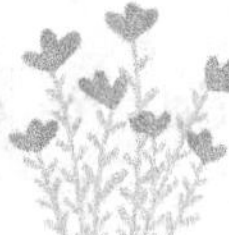

Ingredients:

- 1 lb fresh green beans, trimmed
- 2 tablespoons water
- 1 tablespoon unsalted butter
- 1/2 teaspoon salt
- 1/4 teaspoon black pepper

Is the recipe easy to follow?

63. Steamed Green Beans

Procedure:

1. In a steamer basket set over a saucepan of simmering water, steam the trimmed green beans for 5•7 minutes, or until tender•crisp.

2. Transfer the steamed green beans to a serving bowl.

3. Add the water, unsalted butter, salt, and black pepper to the green beans. Toss gently to coat.

4. Serve the steamed green beans warm.

Nutritional Information (per serving):
Calories: 60
Total Carbs: 6g
Fiber: 3g
Net Carbs: 3g
Protein: 2g
Fat: 3g

This simple steamed green beans recipe is a great way to enjoy this nutritious vegetable. Steaming helps to preserve the green beans' bright color, crisp•tender texture, and fresh flavor. The addition of a small amount of butter, salt, and pepper enhances the natural taste of the green beans without adding too many calories or fat. This side dish is easy to prepare and pairs well with a variety of main courses, from grilled meats to roasted poultry. It's a healthy and versatile option to include in your meal planning.

What are the critical points in the recipe
(e.g., temperature control, timing)?

What is the total cooking time, including prep time?

Prep Time : _______________

Cook Time : _______________

Servings   : _______________

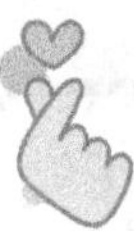

Ingredients:

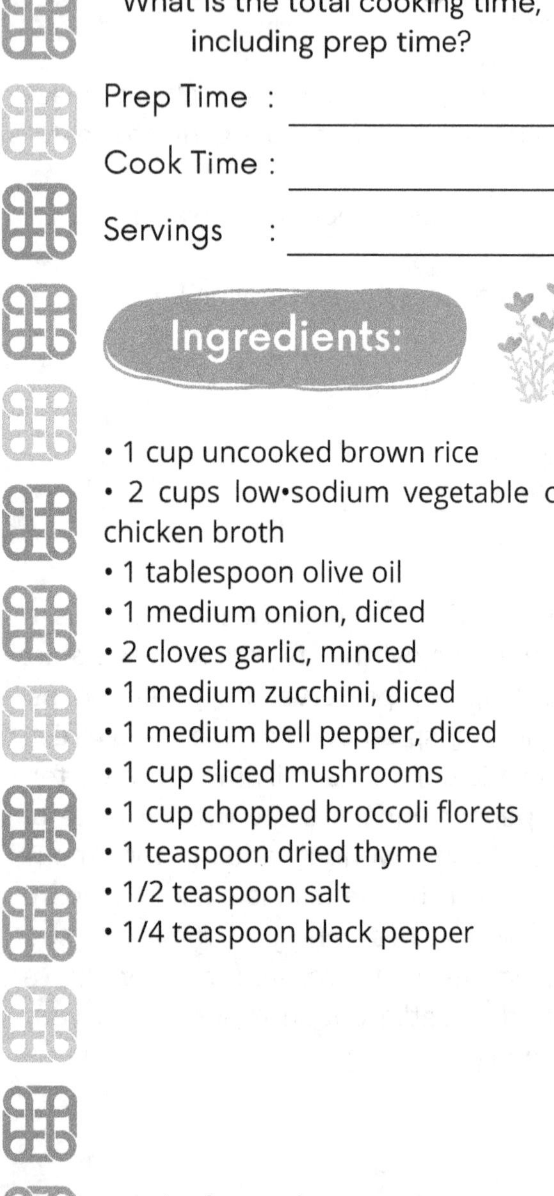

• 1 cup uncooked brown rice
• 2 cups low•sodium vegetable or chicken broth
• 1 tablespoon olive oil
• 1 medium onion, diced
• 2 cloves garlic, minced
• 1 medium zucchini, diced
• 1 medium bell pepper, diced
• 1 cup sliced mushrooms
• 1 cup chopped broccoli florets
• 1 teaspoon dried thyme
• 1/2 teaspoon salt
• 1/4 teaspoon black pepper

Is the recipe easy to follow?

64. Brown Rice with Sautéed Vegetables

Procedure:

1. In a medium saucepan, combine the brown rice and broth. Bring to a boil over high heat. Once boiling, reduce heat to low, cover, and simmer for 25•30 minutes, until rice is tender and liquid is absorbed.

2. In a large skillet, heat the olive oil over medium heat. Add the diced onion and sauté for 3•4 minutes until translucent.

3. Add the minced garlic and sauté for 1 minute until fragrant.

4. Add the diced zucchini, bell pepper, sliced mushrooms, and chopped broccoli florets. Sauté for 5•7 minutes, until vegetables are tender•crisp.

5. Stir in the dried thyme, salt, and black pepper.

6. Fluff the cooked brown rice with a fork and add it to the sautéed vegetables. Toss everything together until well combined.

7. Serve the brown rice and sautéed vegetables warm.

This brown rice and sautéed vegetable dish is a nutritious and flavorful meal. The nutty brown rice provides complex carbohydrates and fiber, while the variety of vegetables add vitamins, minerals, and antioxidants. The simple seasoning of thyme, salt, and pepper complements the natural flavors. This dish is versatile and can be customized with your choice of vegetables.

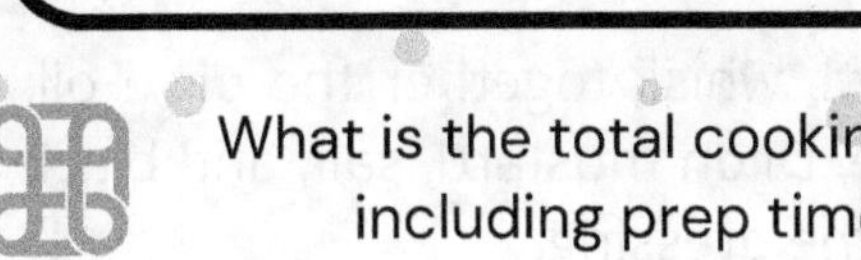

What is the total cooking time, including prep time?

Prep Time : _______________

Cook Time : _______________

Servings : _______________

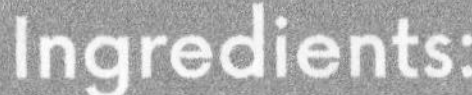

Ingredients:

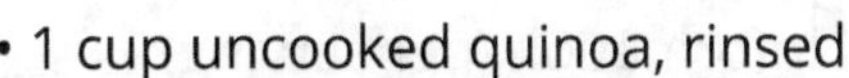

- 1 cup uncooked quinoa, rinsed
- 2 cups low•sodium vegetable or chicken broth
- 1 tablespoon olive oil
- 1 medium onion, diced
- 2 cloves garlic, minced
- 1 cup diced bell pepper (any color)
- 1 cup diced zucchini
- 1 cup diced mushrooms
- 1 teaspoon dried thyme
- 1/2 teaspoon salt
- 1/4 teaspoon black pepper

Is the recipe easy to follow?

65. *Quinoa Pilaf with Vegetables*

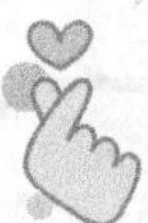

Procedure:

1. In a medium saucepan, combine the rinsed quinoa and broth. Bring to a boil over high heat.

2. Once boiling, reduce the heat to low, cover, and simmer for 15•20 minutes, or until the quinoa is tender and the liquid is absorbed.

3. In a large skillet, heat the olive oil over medium heat. Add the diced onion and sauté for 3•4 minutes until translucent.

4. Add the minced garlic, diced bell pepper, diced zucchini, and diced mushrooms to the skillet. Sauté for 5•7 minutes, until the vegetables are tender.

5. Fluff the cooked quinoa with a fork and add it to the skillet with the sautéed vegetables.

6. Stir in the dried thyme, salt, and black pepper. Toss everything together until well combined.

7. Serve the quinoa pilaf warm.

Nutritional Information (per serving):
Calories: 220
Total Carbs: 32g
Fiber: 5g
Net Carbs: 27g
Protein: 7g
Fat: 7g

This quinoa pilaf is a nutritious and flavorful dish. The quinoa provides a good source of protein and complex carbohydrates, while the variety of vegetables add fiber, vitamins, and minerals. The sautéed onion, garlic, and thyme create a savory base that complements the other ingredients. This quinoa pilaf can be enjoyed as a main course or a side dish, and it's a great option for meal prep.

What is the total cooking time, including prep time?

Prep Time : _______________

Cook Time : _______________

Servings   : _______________

Ingredients:

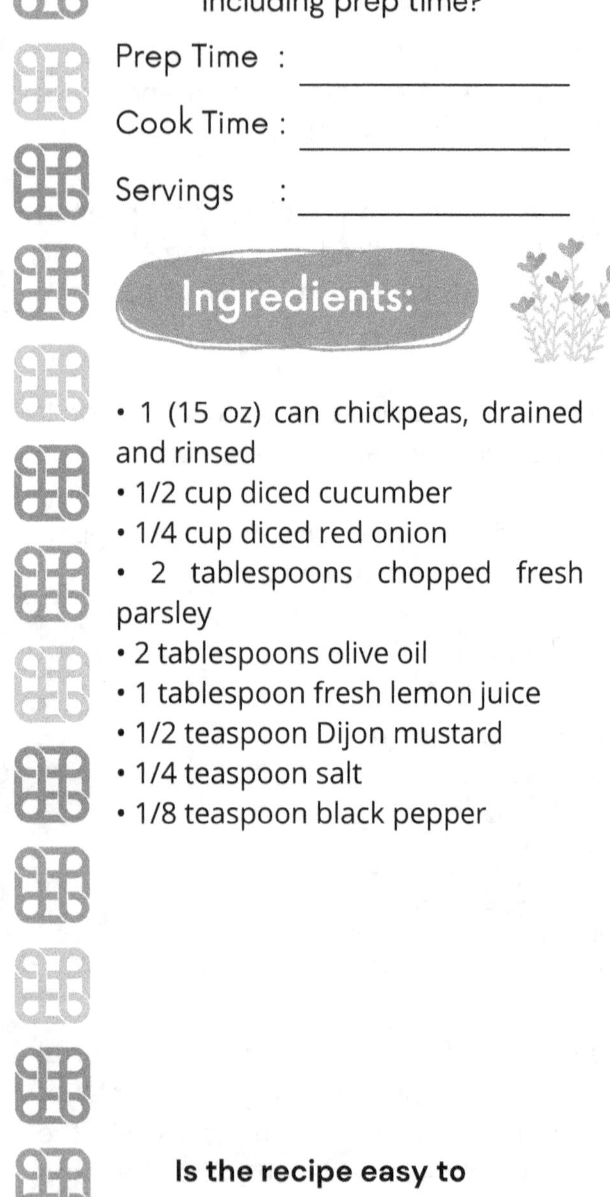

- 1 (15 oz) can chickpeas, drained and rinsed
- 1/2 cup diced cucumber
- 1/4 cup diced red onion
- 2 tablespoons chopped fresh parsley
- 2 tablespoons olive oil
- 1 tablespoon fresh lemon juice
- 1/2 teaspoon Dijon mustard
- 1/4 teaspoon salt
- 1/8 teaspoon black pepper

Is the recipe easy to follow?

66. Chickpea Salad with Lemon and Olive Oil

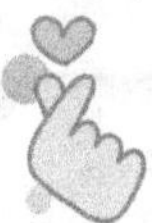

Procedure:

1. In a medium bowl, combine the drained and rinsed chickpeas, diced cucumber, diced red onion, and chopped fresh parsley.

2. In a small bowl, whisk together the olive oil, fresh lemon juice, Dijon mustard, salt, and black pepper to make the dressing.

3. Pour the dressing over the chickpea salad and toss gently to coat.

4. Refrigerate the chickpea salad for at least 30 minutes to allow the flavors to meld.

5. Serve chilled or at room temperature.

Nutritional Information (per serving):
Calories: 150
Total Carbs: 15g
Fiber: 5g
Net Carbs: 10g
Protein: 5g
Fat: 8g

This chickpea salad is a simple, yet flavorful dish. The chickpeas provide a good source of plant·based protein and fiber, while the cucumber, red onion, and parsley add freshness and crunch. The lemon and olive oil dressing adds a bright, tangy flavor that complements the other ingredients. This salad is a great option for a light lunch or a side dish. It's also a versatile recipe that can be customized with your favorite vegetables or herbs.

What is the total cooking time, including prep time?

Prep Time : _______________

Cook Time : _______________

Servings   : _______________

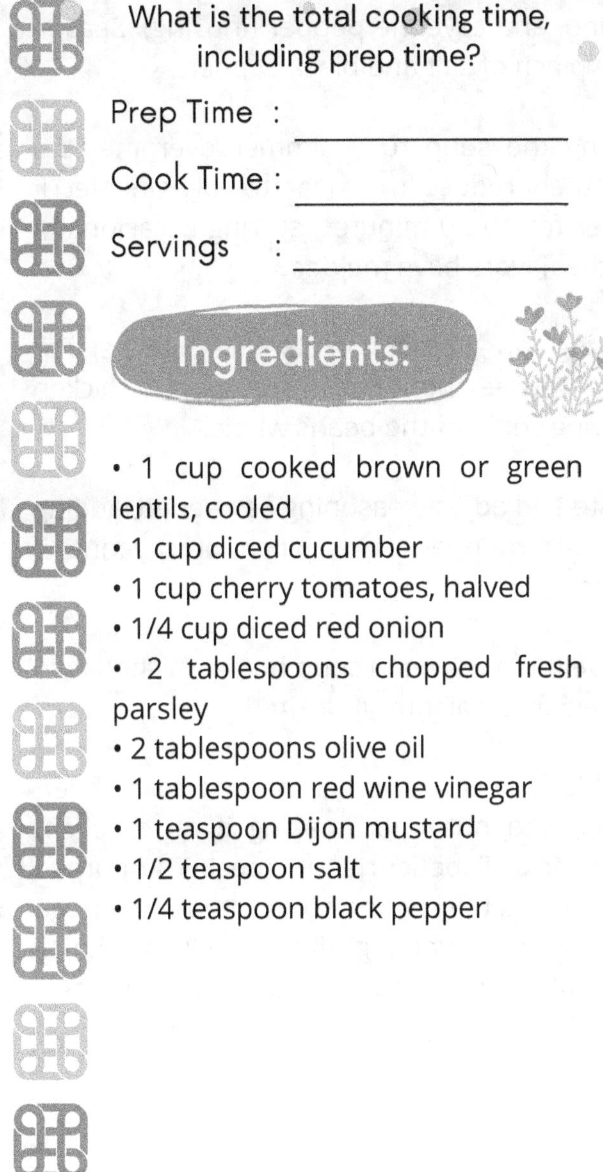

Ingredients:

• 1 cup cooked brown or green lentils, cooled
• 1 cup diced cucumber
• 1 cup cherry tomatoes, halved
• 1/4 cup diced red onion
• 2 tablespoons chopped fresh parsley
• 2 tablespoons olive oil
• 1 tablespoon red wine vinegar
• 1 teaspoon Dijon mustard
• 1/2 teaspoon salt
• 1/4 teaspoon black pepper

Is the recipe easy to follow?

67. Lentil Salad with Cucumbers and Tomatoes

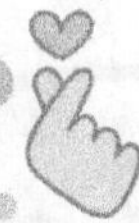

Procedure:

1. In a large bowl, combine the cooked and cooled lentils, diced cucumber, halved cherry tomatoes, diced red onion, and chopped fresh parsley.

2. In a small bowl, whisk together the olive oil, red wine vinegar, Dijon mustard, salt, and black pepper to make the dressing.

3. Pour the dressing over the lentil salad and toss gently to coat.

4. Refrigerate the lentil salad for at least 30 minutes to allow the flavors to meld.

5. Serve chilled or at room temperature.

Nutritional Information (per serving):
Calories: 150
Total Carbs: 16g
Fiber: 6g
Net Carbs: 10g
Protein: 7g
Fat: 8g

This lentil salad is a refreshing and nutritious dish. The lentils provide a good source of plant•based protein and fiber, while the cucumbers, tomatoes, and red onion add crunch and freshness. The simple vinaigrette dressing complements the other ingredients perfectly. This salad can be enjoyed as a light main course or a side dish. It's a great option for meal prep or a potluck, as it holds up well in the refrigerator.

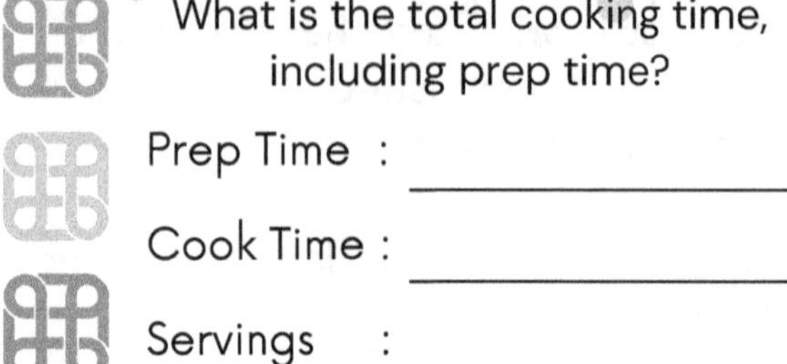

What is the total cooking time, including prep time?

Prep Time : _______________

Cook Time : _______________

Servings : _______________

Ingredients:

- 2 cans (15 oz each) black beans, rinsed and drained
- 1 can (14.5 oz) diced tomatoes, no salt added
- 1 cup low•sodium chicken or vegetable broth
- 1 medium onion, diced
- 2 cloves garlic, minced
- 1 teaspoon ground cumin
- 1 teaspoon dried oregano
- 1/4 teaspoon cayenne pepper (optional, for a little heat)
- Salt and black pepper to taste
- Chopped fresh cilantro for garnish (optional)

Is the recipe easy to follow?

68. Black Bean Soup

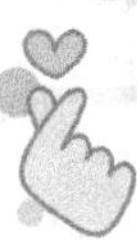

Procedure:

1. In a large saucepan or Dutch oven, combine the rinsed and drained black beans, diced tomatoes, and broth. Stir to mix.

2. Add the diced onion, minced garlic, cumin, oregano, and cayenne pepper (if using). Season with a pinch of salt and black pepper.

3. Bring the soup to a simmer over medium heat, then reduce the heat to low and let it simmer for 15•20 minutes, stirring occasionally, until the flavors have melded.

4. Using an immersion blender or regular blender, puree about half of the soup to thicken it, leaving some of the beans whole.

5. Taste and adjust seasoning as needed, adding more salt, pepper, or a pinch of cayenne if desired.

6. Serve the black bean soup hot, garnished with chopped fresh cilantro if desired.

This black bean soup is packed with fiber, protein, and nutrients, making it an excellent choice for a diabetic•friendly meal. The pureed portion helps thicken the soup without the need for cream or other high•fat ingredients. Enjoy this comforting soup as a main course or as a side dish.

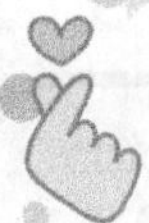

What are the critical points in the recipe (e.g., temperature control, timing)?

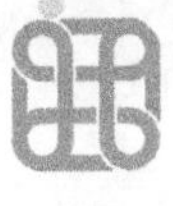

What is the total cooking time, including prep time?

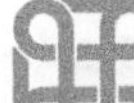
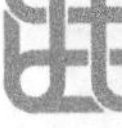
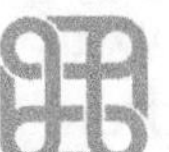

Prep Time : _______________

Cook Time : _______________

Servings   : _______________

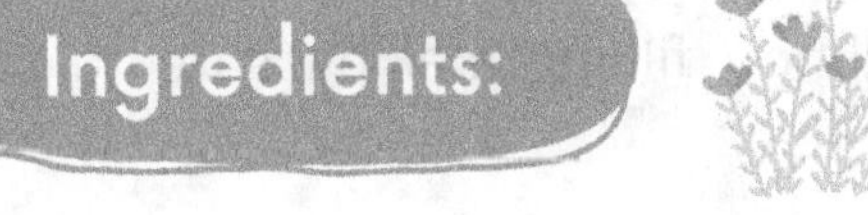

Ingredients:

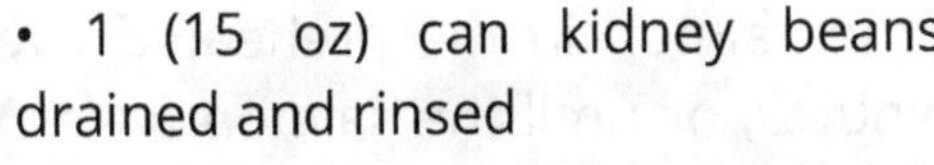
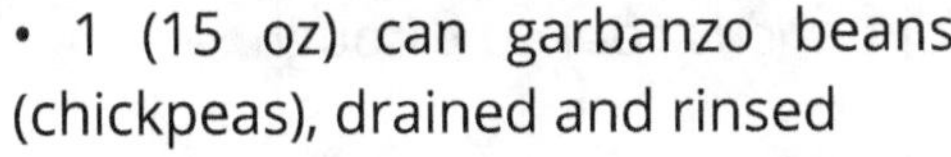

- 1 (15 oz) can kidney beans, drained and rinsed
- 1 (15 oz) can garbanzo beans (chickpeas), drained and rinsed
- 1 (15 oz) can green beans, drained and cut into 1•inch pieces
- 1/2 cup diced red onion
- 1/2 cup apple cider vinegar
- 1/4 cup olive oil
- 2 tablespoons white sugar
- 1 teaspoon salt
- 1/2 teaspoon black pepper

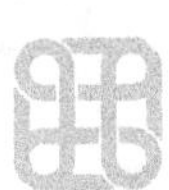
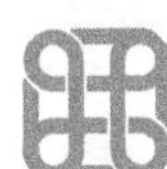
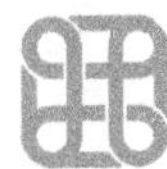

Is the recipe easy to follow?

69. Three•Bean Salad

1. In a large bowl, combine the kidney beans, garbanzo beans, and green beans.

2. Add the diced red onion.

3. In a small bowl, whisk together the apple cider vinegar, olive oil, sugar, salt, and black pepper.

4. Pour the dressing over the bean mixture and stir gently to coat.

5. Cover and refrigerate for at least 2 hours, or up to 3 days, to allow the flavors to meld.

6. Serve chilled or at room temperature.

This classic three•bean salad is a great side dish for picnics, potlucks, or summer barbecues. The combination of kidney beans, garbanzo beans, and green beans with the tangy vinegar dressing is simple but delicious.

What is the total cooking time, including prep time?

Prep Time : _______________

Cook Time : _______________

Servings   : _______________

Ingredients:

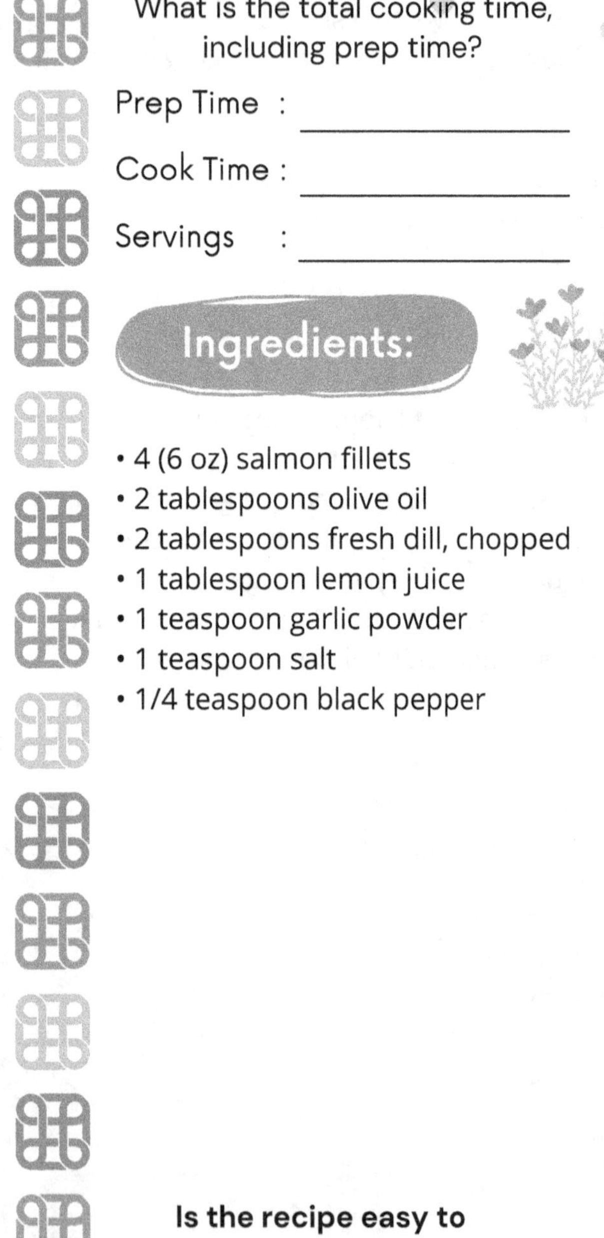

• 4 (6 oz) salmon fillets
• 2 tablespoons olive oil
• 2 tablespoons fresh dill, chopped
• 1 tablespoon lemon juice
• 1 teaspoon garlic powder
• 1 teaspoon salt
• 1/4 teaspoon black pepper

Is the recipe easy to follow?

:) :(

70. Baked Salmon with Dill

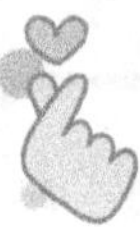

Procedure:

1. Preheat your oven to 400°F (200°C).

2. Line a baking sheet with parchment paper or foil.

3. Place the salmon fillets skin•side down on the prepared baking sheet.

4. In a small bowl, mix together the olive oil, chopped dill, lemon juice, garlic powder, salt, and black pepper.

5. Spoon the dill mixture evenly over the top of the salmon fillets, making sure to coat them completely.

6. Bake the salmon in the preheated oven for 12•15 minutes, or until the salmon flakes easily with a fork and is cooked through.

7. Serve the baked salmon immediately, garnished with additional fresh dill if desired.

This baked salmon with dill is a simple and flavorful way to prepare salmon. The dill, lemon, and garlic complement the rich salmon perfectly. Serve it with roasted vegetables, rice, or a fresh salad for a complete and healthy meal.

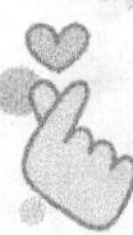

Procedure:

What is the total cooking time,
including prep time?

Prep Time : _______________

Cook Time : _______________

Servings   : _______________

Ingredients:

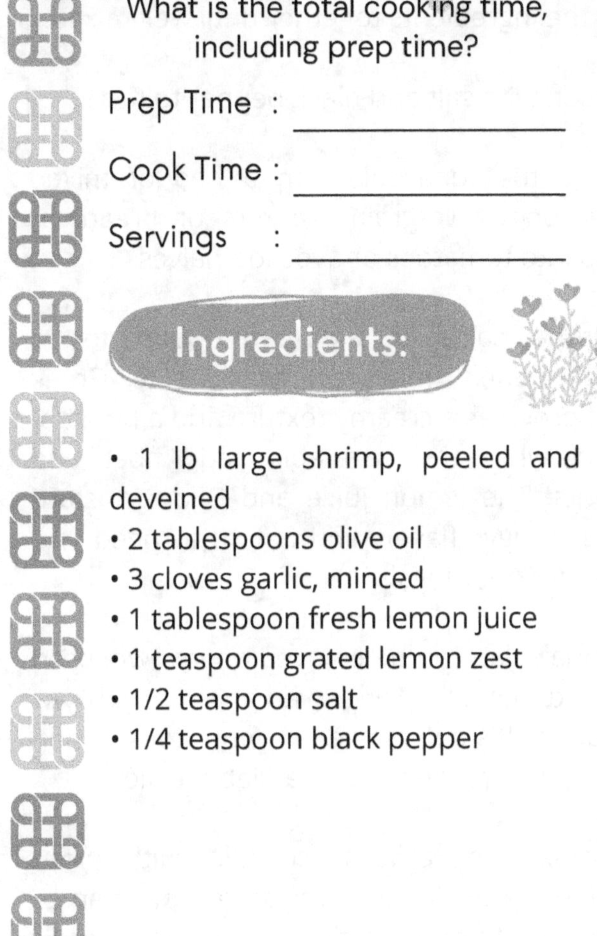

• 1 lb large shrimp, peeled and deveined
• 2 tablespoons olive oil
• 3 cloves garlic, minced
• 1 tablespoon fresh lemon juice
• 1 teaspoon grated lemon zest
• 1/2 teaspoon salt
• 1/4 teaspoon black pepper

Is the recipe easy to follow?

71. *Grilled Shrimp with Garlic and Lemon*

1. In a large bowl, combine the shrimp, olive oil, minced garlic, lemon juice, lemon zest, salt, and black pepper. Toss to coat the shrimp evenly.

2. Preheat your grill or grill pan to medium·high heat.

3. Thread the marinated shrimp onto metal or wooden skewers (if using wooden skewers, soak them in water for 30 minutes first).

4. Grill the shrimp skewers for 2·3 minutes per side, or until the shrimp are opaque and cooked through.

5. Serve the grilled shrimp warm, with any remaining garlic·lemon marinade drizzled over the top.

Nutritional Information (per serving):
Calories: 150
Total Carbs: 2g
Fiber: 0g
Net Carbs: 2g
Protein: 20g
Fat: 8g

This grilled shrimp dish is a simple and flavorful option. The combination of garlic, lemon, and olive oil creates a bright, savory marinade that complements the natural sweetness of the shrimp. Grilling the shrimp adds a nice smoky char and helps to lock in the juices. This dish is low in carbs and high in protein, making it a great choice for a keto or low·carb diet. Serve the grilled shrimp as a main course or as an appetizer.

What is the total cooking time, including prep time?

Prep Time : _________________

Cook Time : _________________

Servings : _________________

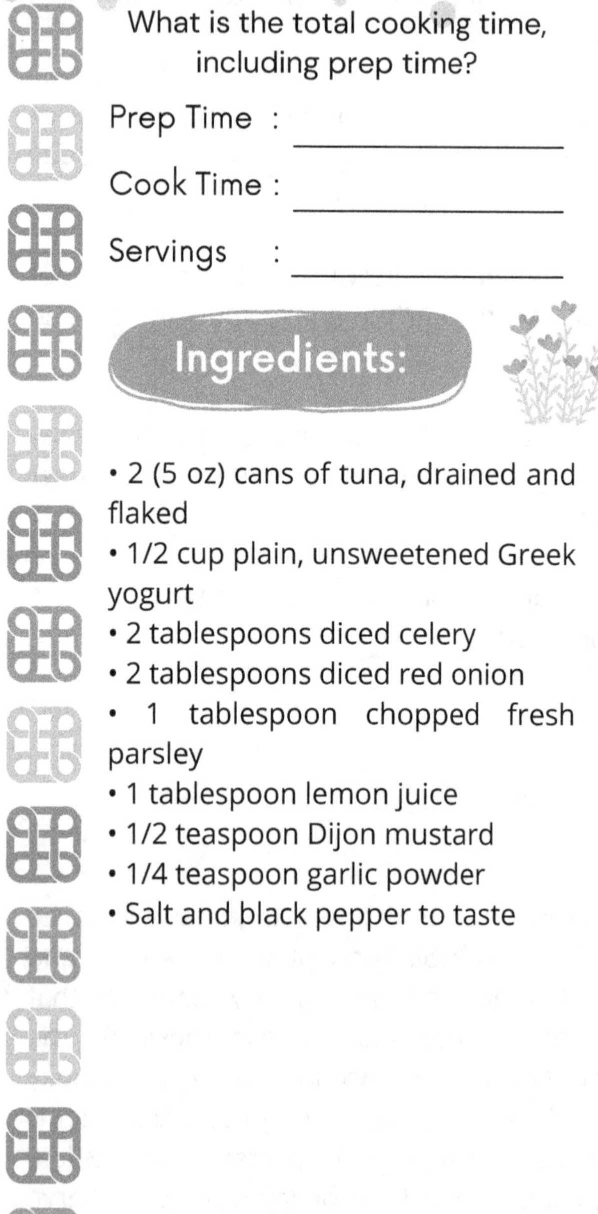

Ingredients:

- 2 (5 oz) cans of tuna, drained and flaked
- 1/2 cup plain, unsweetened Greek yogurt
- 2 tablespoons diced celery
- 2 tablespoons diced red onion
- 1 tablespoon chopped fresh parsley
- 1 tablespoon lemon juice
- 1/2 teaspoon Dijon mustard
- 1/4 teaspoon garlic powder
- Salt and black pepper to taste

Is the recipe easy to follow?

72. *Tuna Salad with Greek Yogurt*

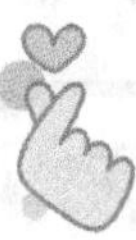

Procedure:

1. In a medium bowl, combine the drained and flaked tuna, Greek yogurt, diced celery, diced red onion, chopped parsley, lemon juice, Dijon mustard, and garlic powder.

2. Stir the ingredients together until well mixed.

3. Season with salt and black pepper to taste.

4. Serve the tuna salad on a bed of mixed greens, on whole•grain crackers or bread, or stuffed into tomatoes or avocado halves.

This tuna salad is a great option for a diabetic•friendly meal or snack. The Greek yogurt provides a creamy texture and a boost of protein, while the vegetables add fiber and nutrients. The lemon juice and Dijon mustard add a tangy flavor without the need for high•sugar dressings.

This tuna salad can be enjoyed on its own, used as a sandwich filling, or served as a dip with raw vegetables. It's a versatile and nutritious option that's perfect for seniors on a diabetic diet.

Remember to always consult with your healthcare provider or a registered dietitian to ensure that this recipe fits within your specific dietary needs and restrictions.

What is the total cooking time, including prep time?

Prep Time : ________________

Cook Time : ________________

Servings : ________________

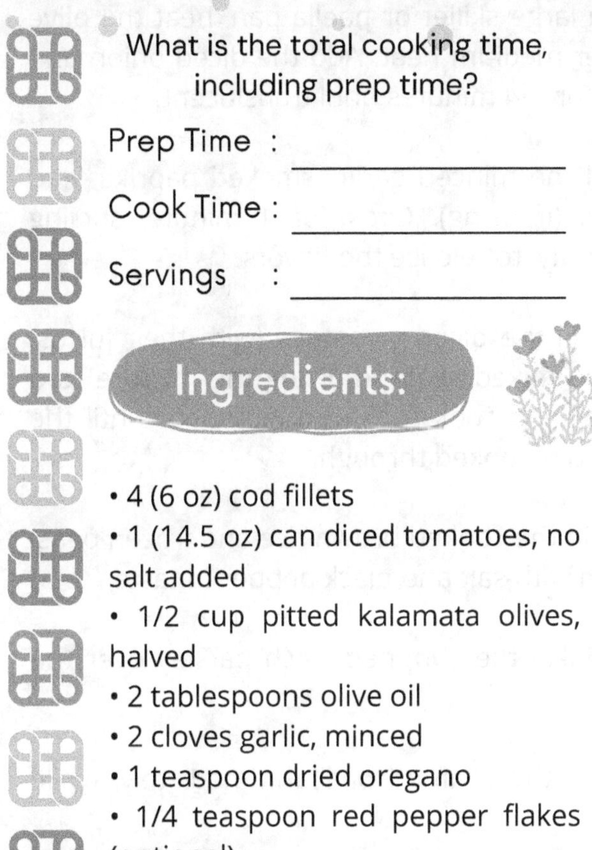

Ingredients:

• 4 (6 oz) cod fillets
• 1 (14.5 oz) can diced tomatoes, no salt added
• 1/2 cup pitted kalamata olives, halved
• 2 tablespoons olive oil
• 2 cloves garlic, minced
• 1 teaspoon dried oregano
• 1/4 teaspoon red pepper flakes (optional)
• Salt and black pepper to taste
• Chopped fresh parsley for garnish (optional)

Is the recipe easy to follow?

73. Baked Cod with Tomatoes and Olives

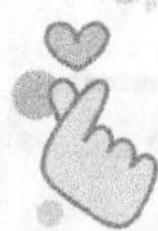

Procedure:

1. Preheat your oven to 400°F (200°C).

2. In a baking dish or oven·safe skillet, combine the diced tomatoes, halved olives, olive oil, minced garlic, dried oregano, and red pepper flakes (if using). Season with a pinch of salt and black pepper. Stir to mix.

3. Place the cod fillets on top of the tomato·olive mixture, making sure they are evenly spaced.

4. Bake the cod in the preheated oven for 15·20 minutes, or until the fish is opaque and flakes easily with a fork.

5. Serve the baked cod immediately, spooning the tomato·olive mixture over the top. Garnish with chopped fresh parsley if desired.

This baked cod dish is a great option for a diabetic·friendly meal. The tomatoes and olives provide a flavorful and nutrient·rich topping for the lean cod, while the baking method keeps the fish moist and tender. Pair this dish with a side of roasted vegetables or a fresh salad for a complete and balanced meal.

Remember to always consult with your healthcare provider or a registered dietitian to ensure that this recipe fits within your specific dietary needs and restrictions.

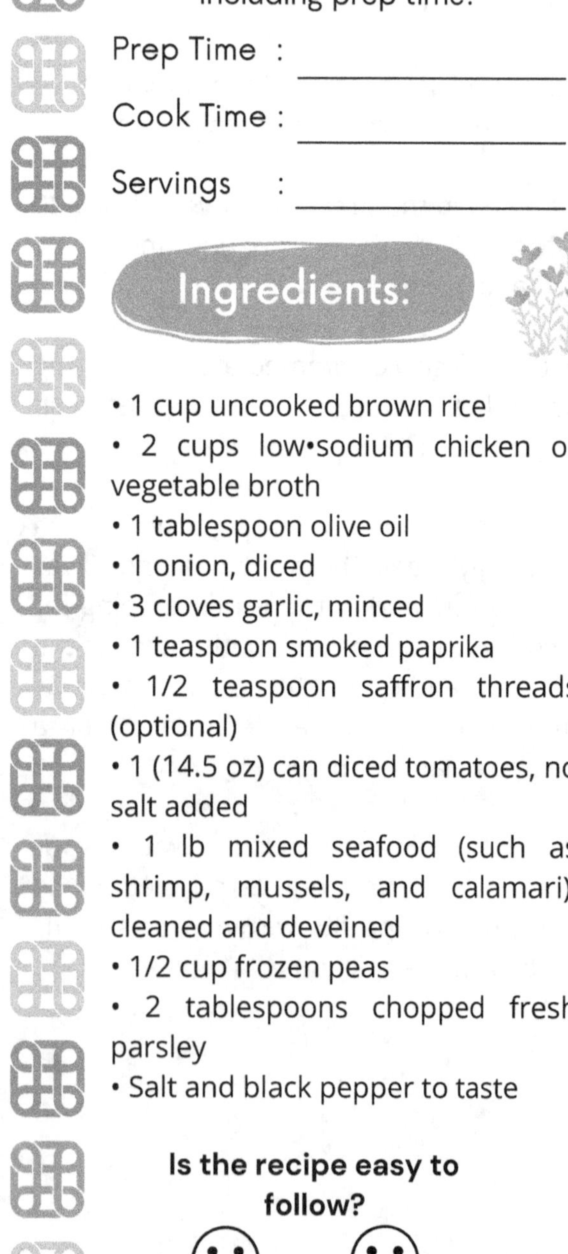

What are the critical points in the recipe (e.g., temperature control, timing)?

What is the total cooking time, including prep time?

Prep Time : _______________

Cook Time : _______________

Servings   : _______________

Ingredients:

• 1 cup uncooked brown rice
• 2 cups low•sodium chicken or vegetable broth
• 1 tablespoon olive oil
• 1 onion, diced
• 3 cloves garlic, minced
• 1 teaspoon smoked paprika
• 1/2 teaspoon saffron threads (optional)
• 1 (14.5 oz) can diced tomatoes, no salt added
• 1 lb mixed seafood (such as shrimp, mussels, and calamari), cleaned and deveined
• 1/2 cup frozen peas
• 2 tablespoons chopped fresh parsley
• Salt and black pepper to taste

Is the recipe easy to follow?

74. Seafood Paella with Brown Rice

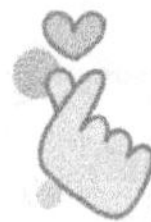

Procedure:

1. Cook the brown rice according to package instructions, using the chicken or vegetable broth instead of water. Set aside.

2. In a large skillet or paella pan, heat the olive oil over medium heat. Add the diced onion and sauté for 3•4 minutes until translucent.

3. Add the minced garlic, smoked paprika, and saffron (if using). Cook for 1 minute, stirring constantly, to release the flavors.

4. Stir in the diced tomatoes (with their juices) and the mixed seafood. Bring the mixture to a simmer and cook for 5•7 minutes, or until the seafood is cooked through.

5. Stir in the cooked brown rice and frozen peas. Season with salt and black pepper to taste.

6. Sprinkle the chopped fresh parsley over the top.

7. Serve the seafood paella immediately, while hot.

This seafood paella with brown rice is a great option for a diabetic•friendly meal for seniors over 50. The brown rice provides a source of complex carbohydrates, while the seafood offers lean protein and healthy omega•3 fatty acids. The vegetables and herbs add fiber, vitamins, and antioxidants.

Remember to always consult with your healthcare provider or a registered dietitian to ensure that this recipe fits within your specific dietary needs and restrictions.

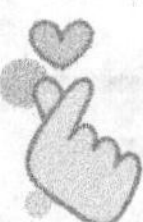

What are the critical points in the recipe (e.g., temperature control, timing)?

What is the total cooking time, including prep time?

Prep Time : ________________

Cook Time : ________________

Servings   : ________________

Ingredients:

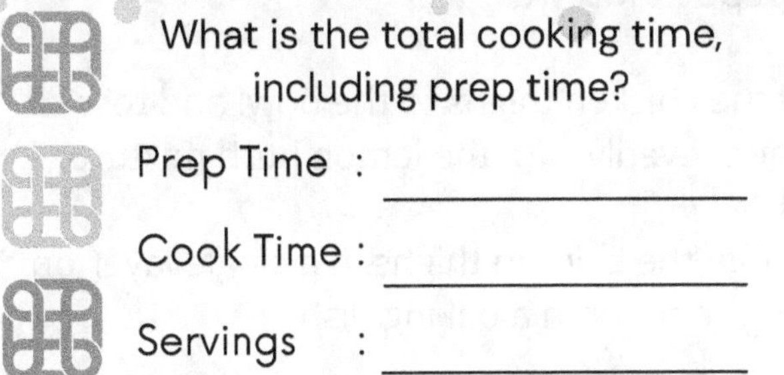

• 2 (6 oz) cans of salmon, drained and flaked
• 1 egg, lightly beaten
• 1/4 cup whole wheat breadcrumbs
• 2 tablespoons chopped fresh parsley
• 1 tablespoon Dijon mustard
• 1 tablespoon lemon juice
• 1/4 teaspoon salt
• 1/4 teaspoon black pepper
• 1 tablespoon olive oil

Side Salad

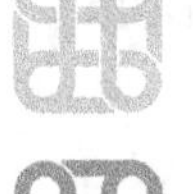

• 5 oz mixed greens
• 1/2 cup cherry tomatoes, halved
• 1/4 cup sliced cucumber
• 2 tablespoons crumbled feta cheese
• 2 tablespoons balsamic vinaigrette

75. Salmon Cakes with a Side Salad

Salmon Cakes:
1. In a medium bowl, combine the flaked salmon, egg, breadcrumbs, parsley, Dijon mustard, lemon juice, salt, and black pepper. Mix well until all the ingredients are evenly distributed.
2. Form the mixture into 4 equal-sized patties.
3. Heat the olive oil in a non-stick skillet over medium heat. Cook the salmon cakes for 3-4 minutes per side, or until golden brown and cooked through.

Side Salad:
1. In a large bowl, combine the mixed greens, cherry tomatoes, sliced cucumber, and crumbled feta cheese.
2. Drizzle the balsamic vinaigrette over the salad and toss gently to coat.

To Serve:
1. Place the salmon cakes on a plate and serve with the side salad.

This meal is a great option for a diabetic-friendly diet for seniors over 50. The salmon cakes provide a lean protein source, while the side salad offers a variety of vegetables and healthy fats from the feta cheese and balsamic vinaigrette. The whole wheat breadcrumbs in the salmon cakes also add some fiber.

Remember to always consult with your healthcare provider or a registered dietitian to ensure that this recipe fits within your specific dietary needs and restrictions.

What is the total cooking time, including prep time?

Prep Time : _________________

Cook Time : _________________

Servings   : _________________

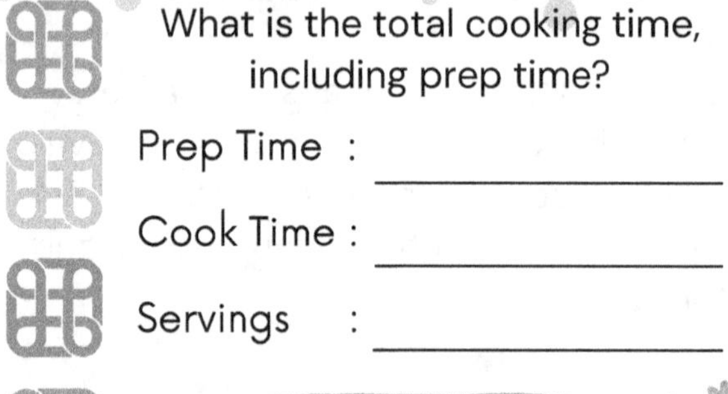

Ingredients:

- 8 boneless, skinless chicken thighs
- 2 tablespoons olive oil
- 2 tablespoons freshly squeezed lemon juice
- 1 tablespoon chopped fresh parsley
- 1 tablespoon chopped fresh thyme
- 2 cloves garlic, minced
- 1 teaspoon grated lemon zest
- 1/2 teaspoon salt
- 1/4 teaspoon black pepper

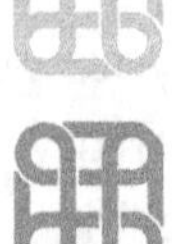

Is the recipe easy to follow?

76. Lemon Herb Chicken Thighs

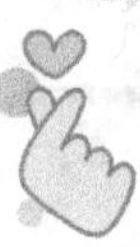

Procedure:

1. Preheat your oven to 400°F (200°C).

2. In a large bowl, combine the olive oil, lemon juice, parsley, thyme, garlic, lemon zest, salt, and black pepper. Mix well.

3. Add the chicken thighs to the bowl and toss to coat them evenly with the lemon herb mixture.

4. Arrange the chicken thighs in a single layer on a baking sheet or in a baking dish.

5. Bake the chicken in the preheated oven for 25•30 minutes, or until the chicken is cooked through and the juices run clear.

6. Optionally, you can broil the chicken for the last 2•3 minutes to get a nice golden•brown color on the top.

7. Serve the lemon herb chicken thighs immediately, garnished with additional fresh parsley or thyme if desired.

This lemon herb chicken thigh recipe is a great option for a diabetic•friendly meal. The chicken thighs are a lean protein source, and the lemon, herbs, and garlic provide plenty of flavor without the need for high•sugar marinades or sauces. Pair this dish with roasted vegetables or a fresh salad for a complete and balanced meal.

Remember to always consult with your healthcare provider or a registered dietitian to ensure that this recipe fits within your specific dietary needs and restrictions.

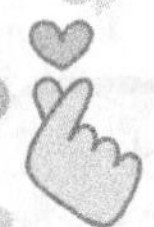

What are the critical points in the recipe (e.g., temperature control, timing)?

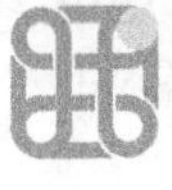

What is the total cooking time, including prep time?

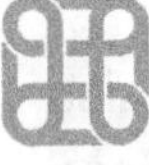

Prep Time : _______________

Cook Time : _______________

Servings   : _______________

Ingredients:

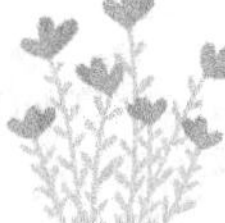

- 1 lb ground turkey
- 1 cup diced onion
- 1 cup diced bell pepper
- 1 cup diced zucchini
- 2 cloves garlic, minced
- 1 egg, lightly beaten
- 1/2 cup whole wheat breadcrumbs
- 2 tablespoons tomato paste
- 1 teaspoon dried oregano
- 1/2 teaspoon salt
- 1/4 teaspoon black pepper

Is the recipe easy to follow?

77. Turkey Meatloaf with Veggies

1. Preheat your oven to 375°F (190°C).

2. In a large bowl, combine the ground turkey, diced onion, diced bell pepper, diced zucchini, minced garlic, beaten egg, whole wheat breadcrumbs, tomato paste, dried oregano, salt, and black pepper. Mix well until all the ingredients are evenly distributed.

3. Lightly grease a 9x5•inch loaf pan. Transfer the turkey mixture to the prepared pan, gently pressing it down to form a compact loaf.

4. Bake the turkey meatloaf in the preheated oven for 50•60 minutes, or until the internal temperature reaches 165°F (75°C).

5. Remove the meatloaf from the oven and let it rest for 5•10 minutes before slicing.

6. Serve the turkey meatloaf warm, with the roasted vegetables on the side.

For the Roasted Vegetables:
- 2 cups diced zucchini
- 2 cups diced bell pepper
- 1 tablespoon olive oil
- 1/2 teaspoon salt
- 1/4 teaspoon black pepper

Toss the diced zucchini and bell pepper with the olive oil, salt, and black pepper. Spread the vegetables on a baking sheet and roast in the oven alongside the meatloaf for 30•40 minutes, or until tender and lightly browned.

This turkey meatloaf with roasted vegetables is a great option for a diabetic•friendly meal. The turkey provides lean protein, while the vegetables add fiber, vitamins, and minerals. The whole wheat breadcrumbs help keep the meatloaf moist and tender.

What is the total cooking time, including prep time?

Prep Time : _______________

Cook Time : _______________

Servings : _______________

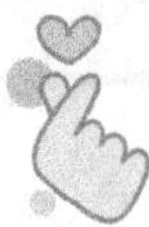

Ingredients:

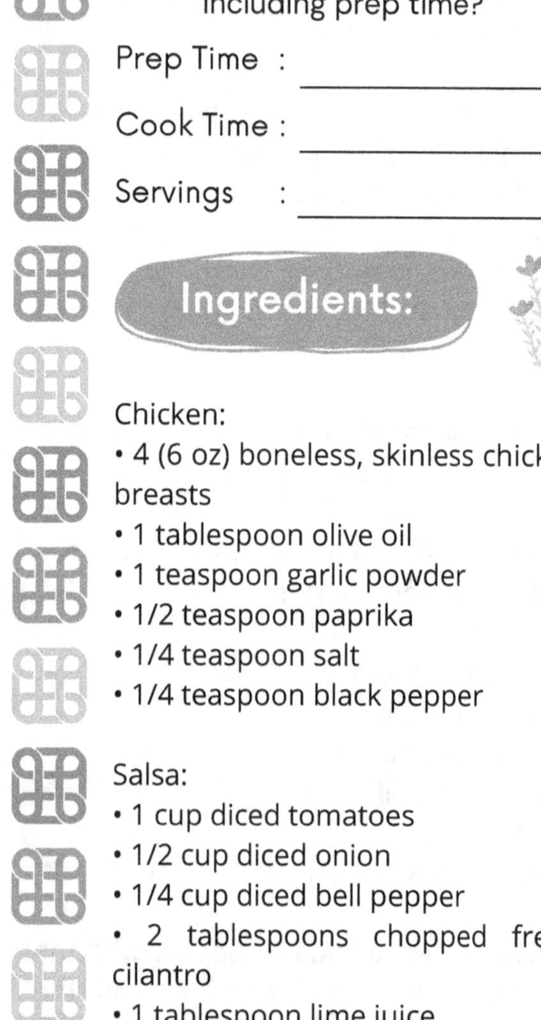

Chicken:
• 4 (6 oz) boneless, skinless chicken breasts
• 1 tablespoon olive oil
• 1 teaspoon garlic powder
• 1/2 teaspoon paprika
• 1/4 teaspoon salt
• 1/4 teaspoon black pepper

Salsa:
• 1 cup diced tomatoes
• 1/2 cup diced onion
• 1/4 cup diced bell pepper
• 2 tablespoons chopped fresh cilantro
• 1 tablespoon lime juice
• 1 clove garlic, minced
• 1/4 teaspoon salt
• 1/4 teaspoon black pepper

Is the recipe easy to follow?

☺   ☹

78. Grilled Chicken Breast with Salsa

Procedure:

1. Preheat your grill or grill pan to medium•high heat.

2. In a small bowl, combine the olive oil, garlic powder, paprika, salt, and black pepper. Rub this seasoning mixture all over the chicken breasts.

3. Grill the chicken for 5•7 minutes per side, or until the internal temperature reaches 165°F (75°C). Transfer the grilled chicken to a plate and let it rest for 5 minutes.

4. In a medium bowl, combine all the salsa ingredients: diced tomatoes, diced onion, diced bell pepper, chopped cilantro, lime juice, minced garlic, salt, and black pepper. Stir to mix well.

5. Serve the grilled chicken breasts topped with the fresh tomato salsa.

This grilled chicken with salsa is a great option for a diabetic•friendly meal. The chicken provides a lean protein source, while the salsa adds a flavorful and nutrient•rich topping. The fresh vegetables and herbs in the salsa provide fiber, vitamins, and antioxidants.

Remember to always consult with your healthcare provider or a registered dietitian to ensure that this recipe fits within your specific dietary needs and restrictions.

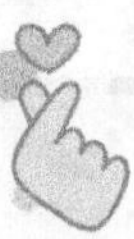

Procedure:

What is the total cooking time,
including prep time?

Prep Time : ______________

Cook Time : ______________

Servings : ______________

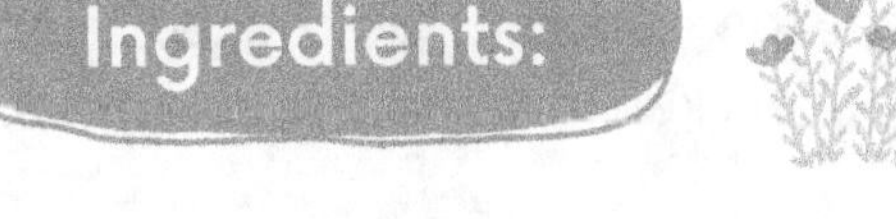

Ingredients:

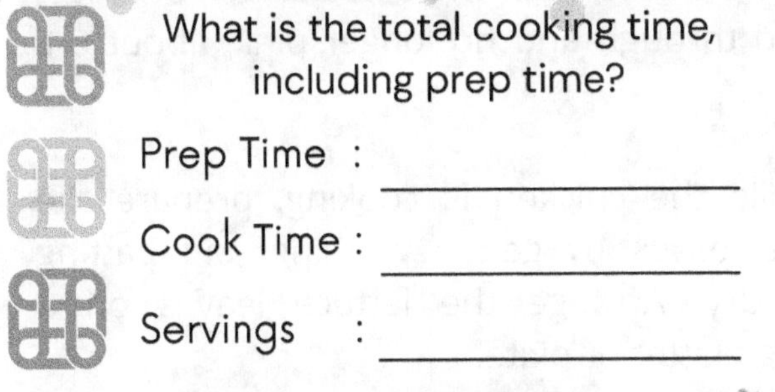

- 8 chicken drumsticks (about 2 lbs)
- 1 tablespoon olive oil
- 1 teaspoon paprika
- 1 teaspoon garlic powder
- 1 teaspoon dried oregano
- 1/2 teaspoon salt
- 1/4 teaspoon black pepper

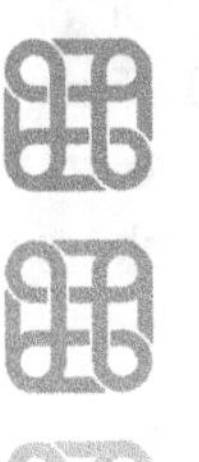

**Is the recipe easy to
follow?**

79. Baked Chicken Drumsticks

1. Preheat your oven to 400°F (200°C). Line a baking sheet with parchment paper or a silicone baking mat.

2. Pat the chicken drumsticks dry with paper towels and place them in a large bowl.

3. In a small bowl, mix together the olive oil, paprika, garlic powder, dried oregano, salt, and black pepper.

4. Pour the seasoning mixture over the chicken drumsticks and toss to coat them evenly.

5. Arrange the seasoned chicken drumsticks on the prepared baking sheet, making sure they are not touching each other.

6. Bake the chicken in the preheated oven for 35·40 minutes, or until the internal temperature reaches 165°F (75°C) when measured with a meat thermometer.

7. Halfway through the baking time, flip the chicken drumsticks to ensure even cooking.

8. Once the chicken is cooked through, remove it from the oven and let it rest for 5 minutes before serving.

Serve the baked chicken drumsticks warm, accompanied by your choice of diabetic·friendly side dishes, such as roasted vegetables, a fresh salad, or a small portion of whole grain rice or quinoa.

This baked chicken drumstick recipe is a great option for a diabetic·friendly meal for seniors over 50. The chicken is a lean protein source, and the simple seasoning adds flavor without the need for high·sugar marinades or sauces.

What are the critical points in the recipe (e.g., temperature control, timing)?

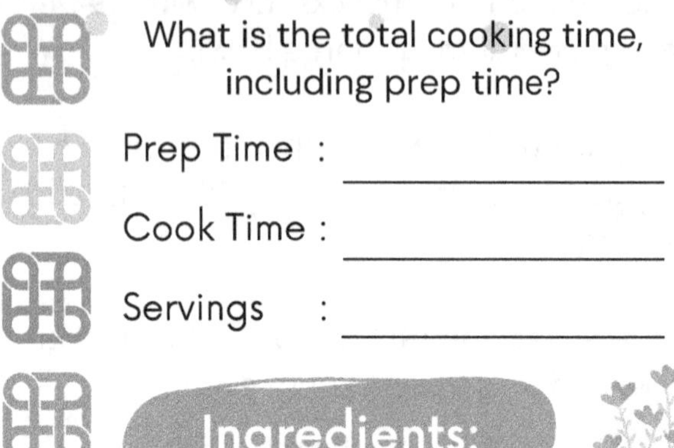

What is the total cooking time, including prep time?

Prep Time : _______________

Cook Time : _______________

Servings : _______________

Ingredients:

- 1 lb boneless, skinless chicken breasts, diced
- 1 tablespoon olive oil
- 1 teaspoon chili powder
- 1/2 teaspoon ground cumin
- 1/4 teaspoon garlic powder
- 1/4 teaspoon onion powder
- Salt and black pepper to taste
- 8•10 large lettuce leaves (such as romaine or bibb)
- Toppings: diced tomatoes, diced onion, shredded low•fat cheddar cheese, diced avocado, salsa, lime wedges

Is the recipe easy to follow?

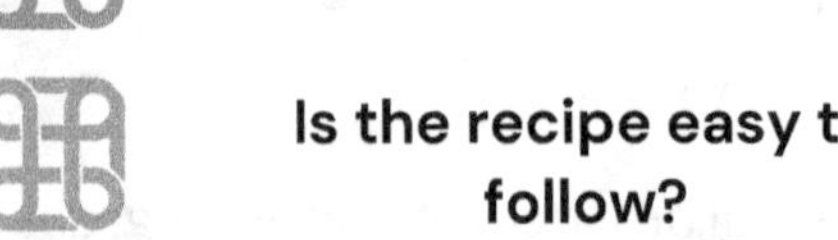

80. Chicken Tacos with Lettuce Wraps

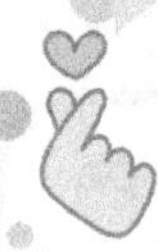

Procedure:

1. In a large skillet, heat the olive oil over medium•high heat. Add the diced chicken and season with the chili powder, cumin, garlic powder, onion powder, salt, and black pepper. Cook the chicken, stirring occasionally, until it is cooked through and no longer pink, about 6•8 minutes.

2. While the chicken is cooking, prepare the lettuce leaves by gently washing and patting them dry. Arrange the lettuce leaves on a serving platter or plate.

3. Once the chicken is cooked, spoon the seasoned chicken into the lettuce leaves.

4. Top the chicken with your desired toppings, such as diced tomatoes, diced onion, shredded low•fat cheddar cheese, diced avocado, and salsa.

5. Serve the chicken tacos with the lettuce wraps immediately, with lime wedges on the side.

This chicken taco recipe is a great option for a diabetic•friendly meal for seniors over 50. The lettuce wraps provide a low•carb alternative to traditional taco shells, and the lean chicken breast, vegetables, and healthy toppings make it a nutritious and balanced meal.

Remember to always consult with your healthcare provider or a registered dietitian to ensure that this recipe fits within your specific dietary needs and restrictions.

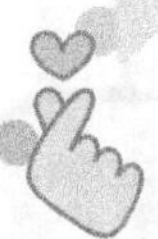

What are the critical points in the recipe (e.g., temperature control, timing)?

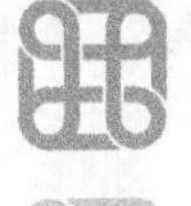

What is the total cooking time, including prep time?

Prep Time : _______________

Cook Time : _______________

Servings : _______________

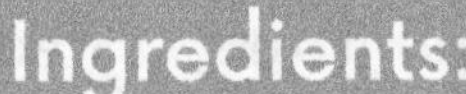 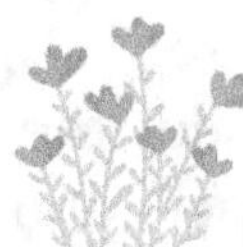

Ingredients:

- 1 lb ground turkey
- 2 tablespoons low•sodium soy sauce
- 1 tablespoon rice vinegar
- 1 teaspoon sesame oil
- 1 teaspoon grated fresh ginger
- 2 cloves garlic, minced
- 1/4 teaspoon red pepper flakes (optional)
- 2 tablespoons olive oil
- 1 cup sliced mushrooms
- 1 cup broccoli florets
- 1 cup sliced bell peppers
- 1 cup shredded cabbage
- 2 green onions, sliced
- 2 cups cooked brown rice

Is the recipe easy to follow?

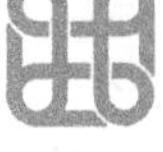  

81. Turkey Stir•Fry with Vegetables

1. In a small bowl, combine the ground turkey, soy sauce, rice vinegar, sesame oil, grated ginger, minced garlic, and red pepper flakes (if using). Mix well and set aside.

2. Heat the olive oil in a large skillet or wok over high heat.

3. Add the sliced mushrooms, broccoli florets, sliced bell peppers, and shredded cabbage to the hot skillet. Stir•fry the vegetables for 4•5 minutes, or until they are crisp•tender.

4. Add the seasoned ground turkey to the skillet and continue to stir•fry for 5•7 minutes, breaking up the turkey with a spatula, until it is cooked through and no longer pink.

5. Stir in the sliced green onions and cook for an additional 1•2 minutes.

6. Serve the turkey stir•fry immediately over the cooked brown rice.

This turkey stir•fry is a great option for a diabetic•friendly meal. The lean ground turkey provides protein, while the variety of vegetables add fiber, vitamins, and minerals. The brown rice serves as a complex carbohydrate source. The soy sauce, ginger, and garlic provide flavor without the need for high•sugar sauces.

Remember to always consult with your healthcare provider or a registered dietitian to ensure that this recipe fits within your specific dietary needs and restrictions.

What is the total cooking time, including prep time?

Prep Time : ___________________

Cook Time : ___________________

Servings   : ___________________

Ingredients:

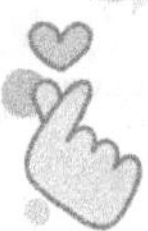

- 1 lb lean beef sirloin or flank steak, thinly sliced
- 2 tablespoons low•sodium soy sauce
- 1 tablespoon rice vinegar
- 1 teaspoon sesame oil
- 2 cloves garlic, minced
- 1 tablespoon grated fresh ginger
- 2 tablespoons olive oil
- 4 cups broccoli florets
- 1 red bell pepper, thinly sliced
- 1 cup sliced mushrooms
- 2 green onions, sliced
- 1/4 teaspoon red pepper flakes (optional)
- 2 cups cooked brown rice

Is the recipe easy to follow?

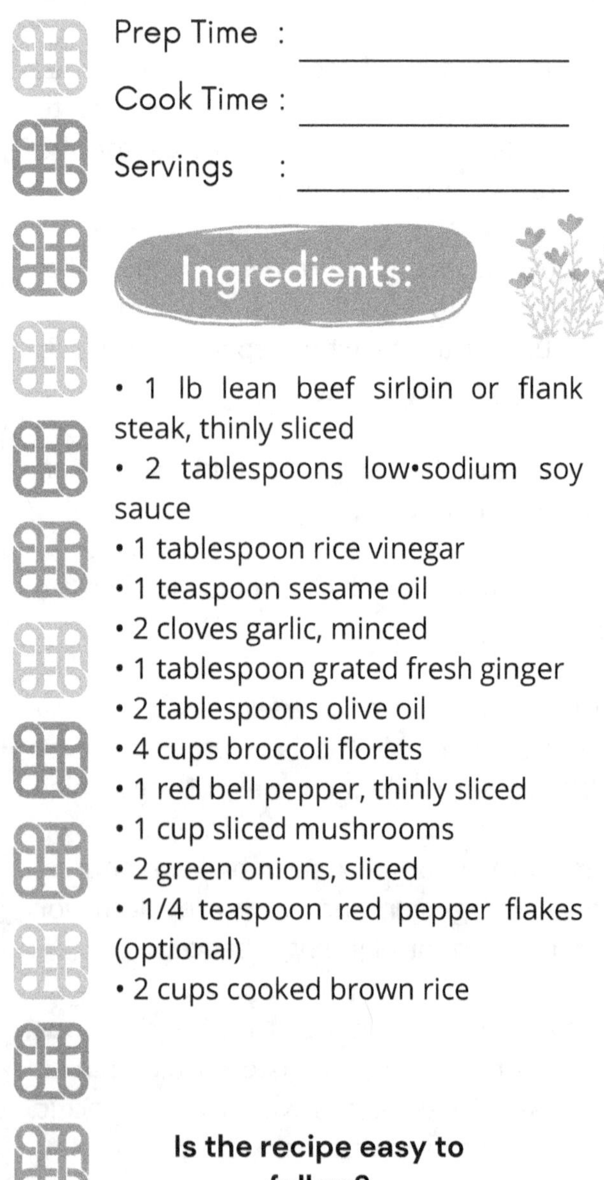

82. Lean Beef Stir•Fry with Broccoli

Procedure:

1. In a medium bowl, combine the sliced beef, soy sauce, rice vinegar, sesame oil, minced garlic, and grated ginger. Toss to coat the beef and let it marinate for 15•20 minutes.

2. Heat the olive oil in a large skillet or wok over high heat.

3. Add the marinated beef to the hot skillet and stir•fry for 3•4 minutes, or until the beef is lightly browned and cooked through. Transfer the beef to a plate and set aside.

4. Add the broccoli florets, sliced red bell pepper, and sliced mushrooms to the skillet. Stir•fry the vegetables for 4•5 minutes, or until they are crisp•tender.

5. Return the cooked beef to the skillet with the vegetables. Add the sliced green onions and red pepper flakes (if using). Stir to combine and heat through, about 2 minutes.

6. Serve the beef and vegetable stir•fry immediately over the cooked brown rice.

This lean beef stir•fry with broccoli is a great option for a diabetic•friendly meal for seniors over 50. The lean beef provides protein, while the broccoli, bell pepper, and mushrooms add fiber, vitamins, and minerals. The brown rice serves as a complex carbohydrate source.

Remember to always consult with your healthcare provider or a registered dietitian to ensure that this recipe fits within your specific dietary needs and restrictions.

What is the total cooking time, including prep time?

Prep Time : _______________

Cook Time : _______________

Servings   : _______________

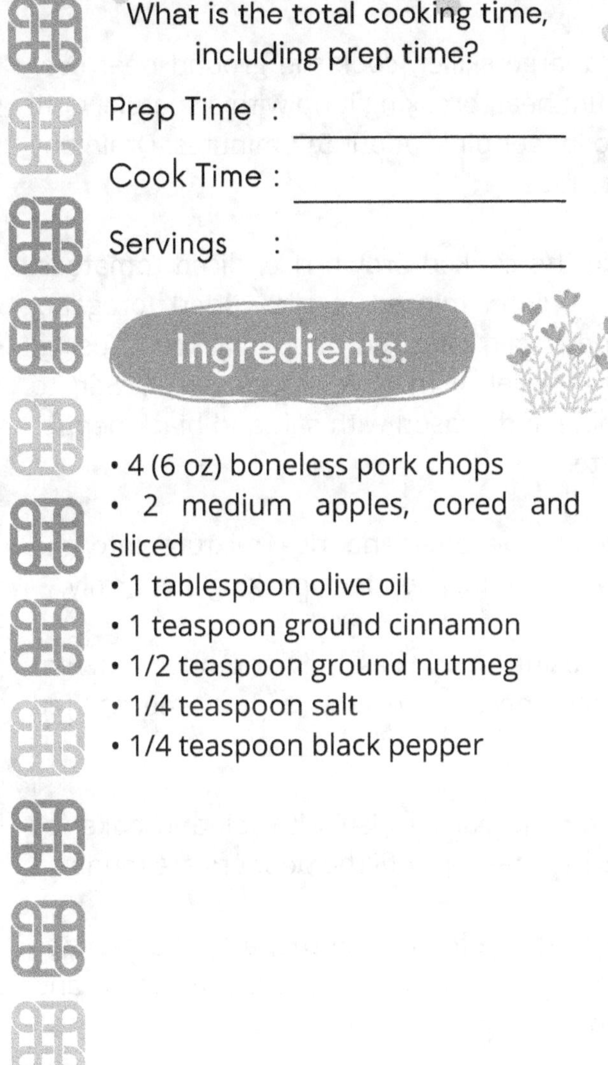

Ingredients:

- 4 (6 oz) boneless pork chops
- 2 medium apples, cored and sliced
- 1 tablespoon olive oil
- 1 teaspoon ground cinnamon
- 1/2 teaspoon ground nutmeg
- 1/4 teaspoon salt
- 1/4 teaspoon black pepper

Is the recipe easy to follow?

83. Baked Pork Chops with Apples

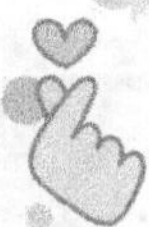

Procedure:

1. Preheat your oven to 400°F (200°C).

2. In a large bowl, combine the sliced apples, olive oil, cinnamon, nutmeg, salt, and black pepper. Toss to coat the apples evenly.

3. Arrange the pork chops in a baking dish or on a rimmed baking sheet. Spread the seasoned apple slices around and on top of the pork chops.

4. Bake the pork chops and apples in the preheated oven for 25·30 minutes, or until the pork chops are cooked through and reach an internal temperature of 145°F (63°C).

5. Remove the baked pork chops and apples from the oven and let them rest for 5 minutes before serving.

6. Serve the pork chops with the baked apples on the side.

This baked pork chops with apples recipe is a great option for a diabetic·friendly meal for seniors over 50. The pork chops provide a lean protein source, while the apples add natural sweetness and fiber. The cinnamon and nutmeg add warmth and flavor without the need for high·sugar sauces or marinades.

Remember to always consult with your healthcare provider or a registered dietitian to ensure that this recipe fits within your specific dietary needs and restrictions.

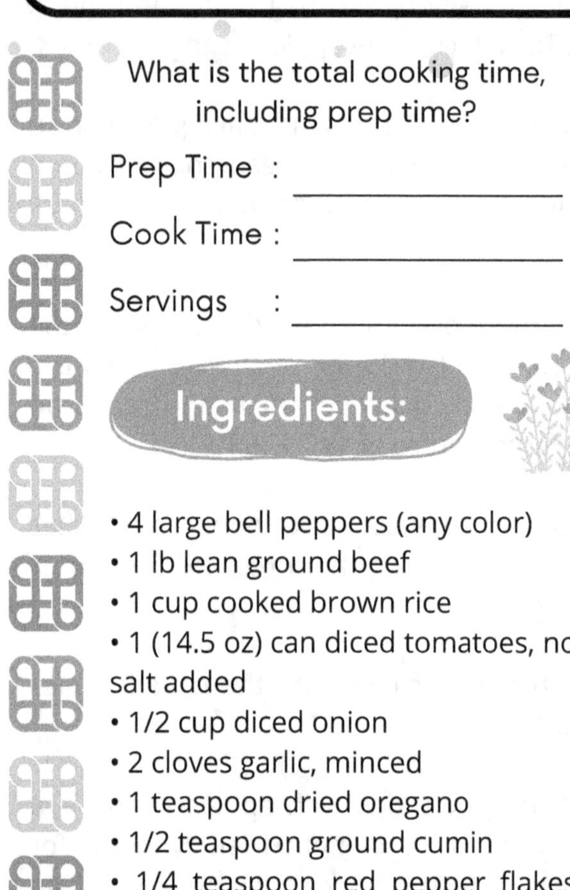

What is the total cooking time, including prep time?

Prep Time : ______________

Cook Time : ______________

Servings   : ______________

Ingredients:

- 4 large bell peppers (any color)
- 1 lb lean ground beef
- 1 cup cooked brown rice
- 1 (14.5 oz) can diced tomatoes, no salt added
- 1/2 cup diced onion
- 2 cloves garlic, minced
- 1 teaspoon dried oregano
- 1/2 teaspoon ground cumin
- 1/4 teaspoon red pepper flakes (optional)
- Salt and black pepper to taste
- 1/2 cup shredded low•fat cheddar cheese (optional)

Is the recipe easy to follow?

84. Stuffed Peppers with Ground Beef

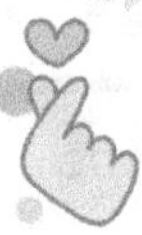

Procedure:

1. Preheat your oven to 375°F (190°C).

2. Cut the tops off the bell peppers and remove the seeds and membranes. Place the peppers in a baking dish and set aside.

3. In a large skillet, cook the ground beef over medium heat, breaking it up with a spatula, until it's no longer pink, about 5•7 minutes. Drain any excess fat.

4. Add the cooked brown rice, diced tomatoes, diced onion, minced garlic, dried oregano, ground cumin, and red pepper flakes (if using) to the skillet with the ground beef. Stir to combine and season with salt and black pepper to taste.

5. Spoon the beef and rice mixture into the hollowed•out bell peppers, packing it in firmly.

6. If using, sprinkle the shredded low•fat cheddar cheese over the top of the stuffed peppers.

7. Cover the baking dish with foil and bake for 30•35 minutes, or until the peppers are tender.

8. Remove the foil during the last 5•10 minutes of baking to allow the cheese to melt and brown, if using.

9. Serve the stuffed peppers warm.

This stuffed pepper recipe is a great option for a diabetic•friendly meal. The bell peppers provide fiber, while the lean ground beef and brown rice offer protein and complex carbohydrates. The low•fat cheese is optional, but it can add a nice creamy texture if desired.

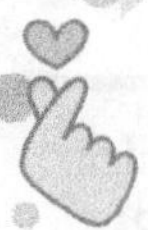

Procedure:

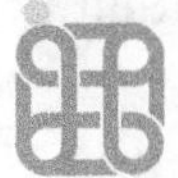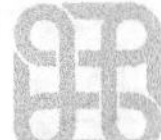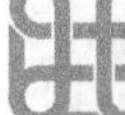

What is the total cooking time, including prep time?

Prep Time : ________________

Cook Time : ________________

Servings : ________________

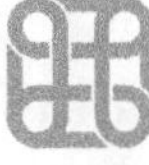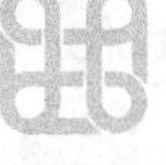

Ingredients:

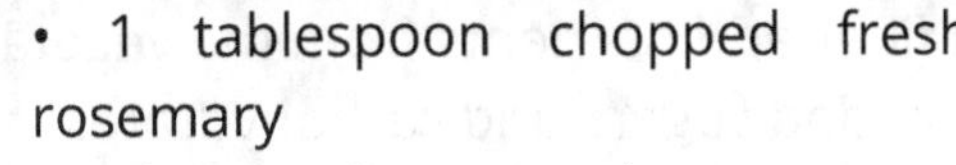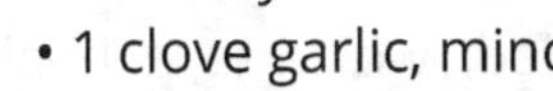

- 4 (4 oz) lamb chops
- 1 tablespoon olive oil
- 1 tablespoon chopped fresh rosemary
- 1 clove garlic, minced
- 1/2 teaspoon salt
- 1/4 teaspoon black pepper

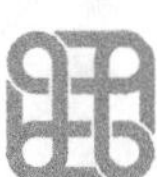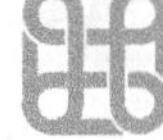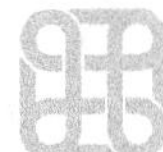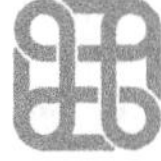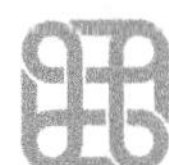

Is the recipe easy to follow?

85. *Grilled Lamb Chops with Rosemary*

1. Preheat your grill or grill pan to medium•high heat.

2. In a small bowl, combine the olive oil, chopped rosemary, minced garlic, salt, and black pepper. Mix well to create a marinade.

3. Rub the marinade all over the lamb chops, making sure to coat them evenly on both sides.

4. Grill the lamb chops for 3•4 minutes per side, or until they reach the desired level of doneness. For medium•rare, the internal temperature should reach 130•135°F (54•57°C).

5. Transfer the grilled lamb chops to a plate and let them rest for 5 minutes before serving.

Serve the grilled lamb chops warm, accompanied by your choice of diabetic•friendly side dishes, such as:

- Roasted vegetables (e.g., zucchini, bell peppers, onions)
- A fresh salad with a light vinaigrette dressing
- Steamed broccoli or green beans
- Quinoa or brown rice

This grilled lamb chops with rosemary recipe is a great option for a diabetic•friendly meal for seniors over 50. Lamb is a lean protein source, and the rosemary and garlic add flavor without the need for high•sugar marinades or sauces.

Remember to always consult with your healthcare provider or a registered dietitian to ensure that this recipe fits within your specific dietary needs and restrictions.

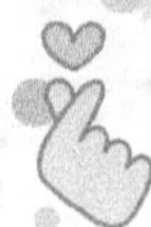

Procedure:

What is the total cooking time, including prep time?

Prep Time : _______________

Cook Time : _______________

Servings   : _______________

Ingredients:

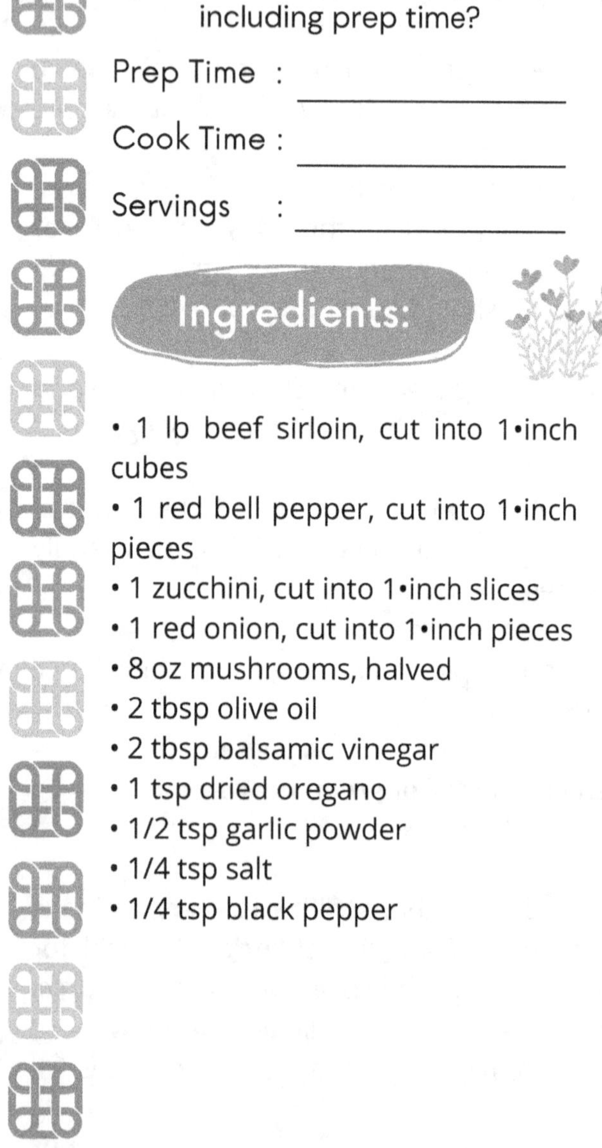

• 1 lb beef sirloin, cut into 1•inch cubes
• 1 red bell pepper, cut into 1•inch pieces
• 1 zucchini, cut into 1•inch slices
• 1 red onion, cut into 1•inch pieces
• 8 oz mushrooms, halved
• 2 tbsp olive oil
• 2 tbsp balsamic vinegar
• 1 tsp dried oregano
• 1/2 tsp garlic powder
• 1/4 tsp salt
• 1/4 tsp black pepper

1. Preheat grill or grill pan to medium•high heat.
2. In a large bowl, combine the beef, bell pepper, zucchini, onion, and mushrooms.
3. In a small bowl, whisk together the olive oil, balsamic vinegar, oregano, garlic powder, salt, and black pepper.
4. Pour the marinade over the beef and vegetables and toss to coat evenly.
5. Thread the beef and vegetables onto skewers, alternating the ingredients.
6. Grill the kebabs for 12•15 minutes, turning occasionally, until the beef is cooked through and the vegetables are tender.
7. Serve immediately.

This recipe is suitable for a diabetic diet for seniors over 50 because it is:
• High in protein from the beef
• Rich in fiber and nutrients from the vegetables
• Low in added sugars and carbohydrates
• Grilled instead of fried, which is a healthier cooking method

The portion size and nutrient balance make this a great option for a diabetic•friendly meal.

Is the recipe easy to follow?

86. Beef and Vegetable Kebabs

What are the critical points in the recipe (e.g., temperature control, timing)?

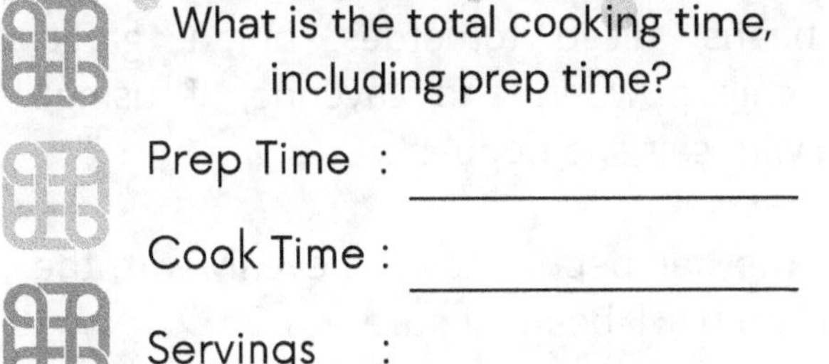

What is the total cooking time, including prep time?

Prep Time : _________________

Cook Time : _________________

Servings   : _________________

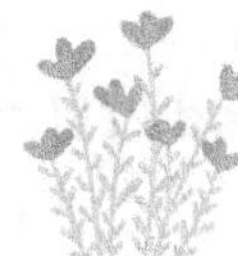

Ingredients:

- 3•4 lb pork shoulder or butt, trimmed of excess fat
- 1 tbsp smoked paprika
- 1 tbsp brown sugar
- 1 tsp garlic powder
- 1 tsp onion powder
- 1 tsp salt
- 1/2 tsp black pepper
- 1 cup chicken or beef broth
- 1 medium head green cabbage, shredded
- 1 cup shredded carrots
- 1/2 cup thinly sliced red onion
- 1/4 cup apple cider vinegar
- 2 tbsp olive oil
- 1 tbsp Dijon mustard
- 1 tsp sugar
- Salt and pepper to taste

Is the recipe easy to follow?

87. Slow•Cooked Pulled Pork with Cabbage Slaw

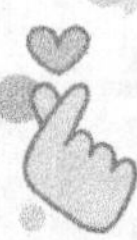

Procedure:

1. In a small bowl, mix together the smoked paprika, brown sugar, garlic powder, onion powder, salt and pepper. Rub this seasoning mix all over the pork.

2. Place the pork in a slow cooker and pour the broth around the sides. Cover and cook on low for 8•10 hours, until the pork is very tender and shreds easily with a fork.

3. Remove the pork from the slow cooker and shred it using two forks. Discard any excess fat.

4. In a large bowl, combine the shredded cabbage, carrots, and red onion.

5. In a small bowl, whisk together the apple cider vinegar, olive oil, Dijon mustard, and sugar. Season with salt and pepper.

6. Pour the dressing over the cabbage slaw and toss to coat evenly.

7. Serve the pulled pork on buns or rolls, topped with the cabbage slaw. Enjoy!

What is the total cooking time, including prep time?

Prep Time : ______________

Cook Time : ______________

Servings : ______________

Ingredients:

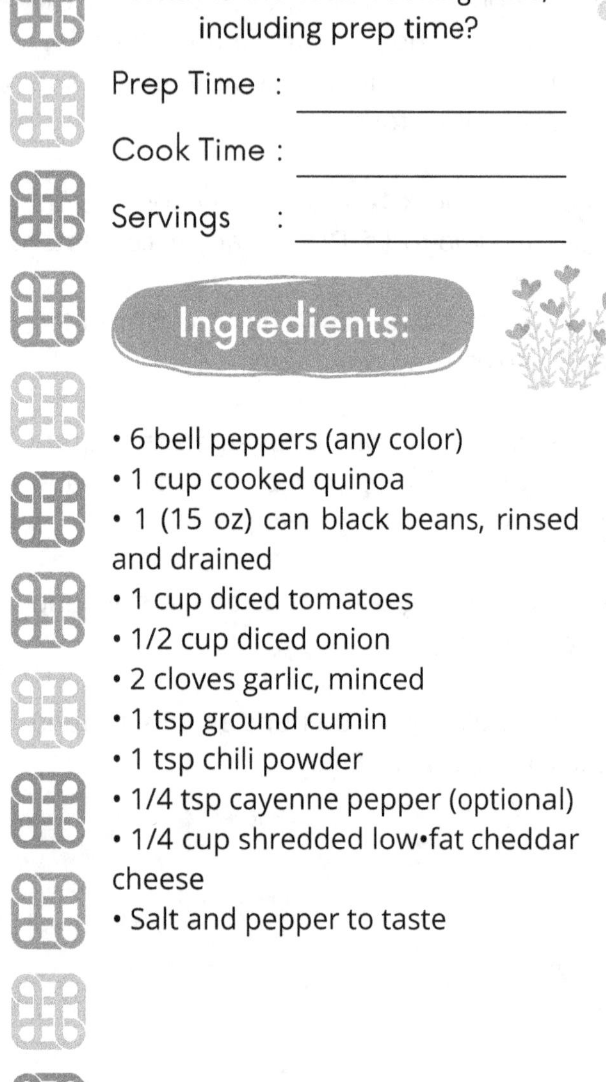

- 6 bell peppers (any color)
- 1 cup cooked quinoa
- 1 (15 oz) can black beans, rinsed and drained
- 1 cup diced tomatoes
- 1/2 cup diced onion
- 2 cloves garlic, minced
- 1 tsp ground cumin
- 1 tsp chili powder
- 1/4 tsp cayenne pepper (optional)
- 1/4 cup shredded low•fat cheddar cheese
- Salt and pepper to taste

Is the recipe easy to follow?

88. Black Bean and Quinoa Stuffed Peppers

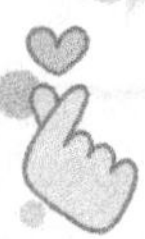

Procedure:

1. Preheat oven to 375°F. Cut the tops off the bell peppers and remove the seeds and membranes. Place the peppers in a baking dish.

2. In a large bowl, combine the cooked quinoa, black beans, diced tomatoes, onion, garlic, cumin, chili powder, and cayenne (if using). Season with salt and pepper.

3. Stuff the bell pepper cavities evenly with the quinoa and black bean mixture.

4. Top each stuffed pepper with a sprinkle of the shredded cheddar cheese.

5. Cover the baking dish with foil and bake for 30•35 minutes, until the peppers are tender.

6. Remove the foil and bake for an additional 5•10 minutes to lightly brown the tops.

7. Serve the stuffed peppers warm.

This recipe is diabetes•friendly as it is high in fiber, protein, and complex carbs from the quinoa and black beans, while being low in saturated fat and added sugars. The bell peppers also provide important vitamins and minerals. Enjoy!

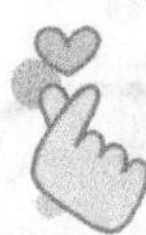

Procedure:

1. In a small bowl, combine the soy sauce, rice vinegar, and sesame oil. Add the cubed tofu and toss gently to coat. Set aside.

2. Heat the olive oil in a large skillet or wok over medium•high heat. Add the garlic and ginger and cook for 1 minute, stirring constantly.

3. Add the bell pepper, broccoli, mushrooms, snow/snap peas, and cabbage. Stir•fry for 3•4 minutes until the vegetables are crisp•tender.

4. Add the marinated tofu and its sauce to the skillet. Stir to combine.

5. In a small bowl, whisk together the vegetable broth and cornstarch. Pour this mixture into the skillet and let it simmer for 2•3 minutes until the sauce has thickened.

6. Remove from heat and stir in the sliced green onions. Season with salt and pepper to taste.

7. Serve the vegetable stir•fry immediately, over steamed brown rice or quinoa if desired.

This stir•fry is diabetes•friendly as it is high in fiber, protein, and complex carbs, while being low in saturated fat and added sugars. The variety of vegetables provide important vitamins, minerals, and antioxidants.

What are the critical points in the recipe (e.g., temperature control, timing)?

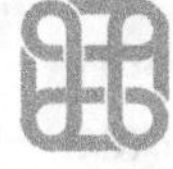
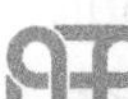
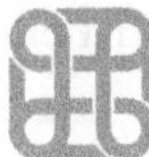

What is the total cooking time, including prep time?

Prep Time : _______________

Cook Time : _______________

Servings   : _______________

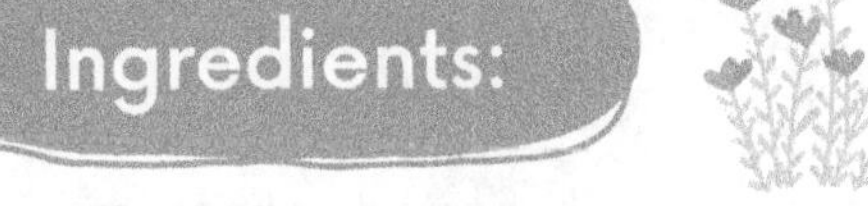

Ingredients:

- 1 block (14 oz) extra•firm tofu, drained and cubed
- 2 tbsp low•sodium soy sauce
- 1 tbsp rice vinegar
- 1 tsp sesame oil
- 1 tbsp olive oil
- 3 cloves garlic, minced
- 1 tbsp grated fresh ginger
- 1 red bell pepper, sliced
- 1 cup broccoli florets
- 1 cup sliced mushrooms
- 1 cup snow peas or snap peas
- 1 cup shredded cabbage
- 2 green onions, sliced
- 1/4 cup low•sodium vegetable or chicken broth
- 1 tsp cornstarch
- Salt and pepper to taste

Is the recipe easy to follow?

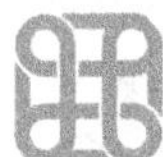

89. Vegetable Stir•Fry with Tofu

What is the total cooking time,
including prep time?

Prep Time : _______________

Cook Time : _______________

Servings   : _______________

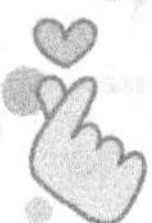

Ingredients:

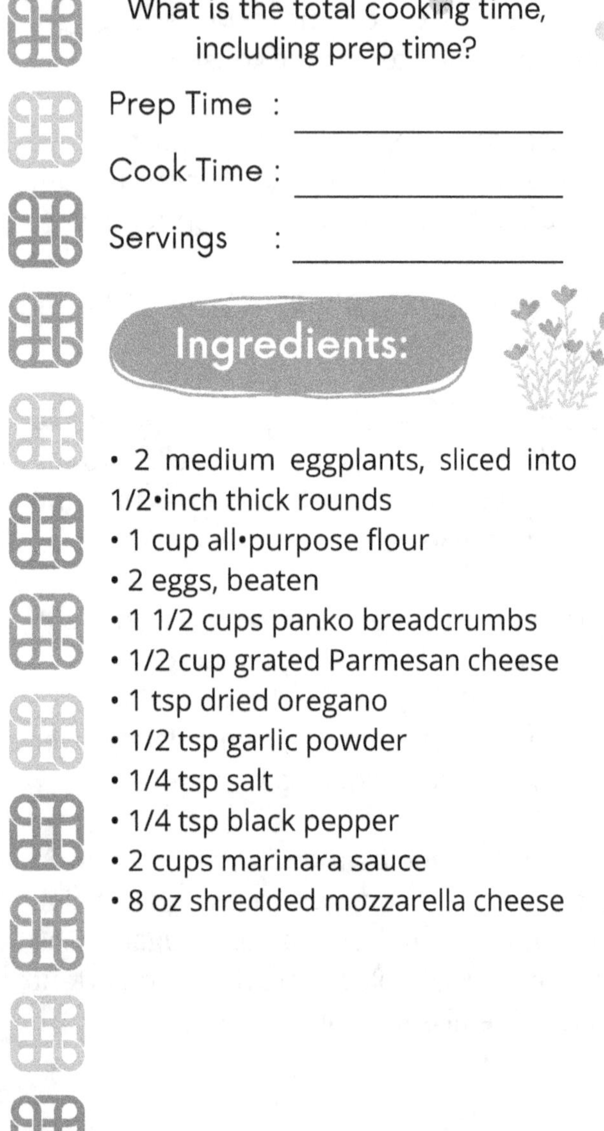

• 2 medium eggplants, sliced into 1/2•inch thick rounds
• 1 cup all•purpose flour
• 2 eggs, beaten
• 1 1/2 cups panko breadcrumbs
• 1/2 cup grated Parmesan cheese
• 1 tsp dried oregano
• 1/2 tsp garlic powder
• 1/4 tsp salt
• 1/4 tsp black pepper
• 2 cups marinara sauce
• 8 oz shredded mozzarella cheese

Is the recipe easy to follow?

90. Eggplant Parmesan

Procedure:

1. Preheat oven to 375°F. Line a baking sheet with parchment paper.

2. Set up a breading station with 3 shallow dishes • one with the flour, one with the beaten eggs, and one with the panko, Parmesan, oregano, garlic powder, salt and pepper mixed together.

3. Dip the eggplant slices first in the flour, shaking off any excess. Then dip in the egg, allowing any excess to drip off. Finally, coat the eggplant in the panko mixture, pressing gently to adhere.

4. Arrange the breaded eggplant slices in a single layer on the prepared baking sheet.

5. Bake for 20 minutes, flip the slices, then bake for another 15•20 minutes until golden brown.

6. Spread 1 cup of the marinara sauce in the bottom of a 9x13 inch baking dish. Arrange the baked eggplant slices in a single layer on top.

7. Top the eggplant with the remaining 1 cup of marinara sauce and the shredded mozzarella cheese.

8. Bake for 20•25 minutes, until the cheese is melted and bubbly.

9. Let stand for 5 minutes before serving. Enjoy!

This eggplant parmesan is a delicious and comforting vegetarian dish. The breaded and baked eggplant slices provide a nice texture contrast to the melty cheese and marinara sauce.

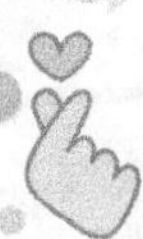

Procedure:

1. In a large skillet or pot, heat the olive oil over medium heat. Add the onion and sauté for 3•4 minutes until translucent.

2. Add the garlic, ginger, curry powder, cumin, coriander, and cayenne (if using). Cook for 1 minute, stirring constantly, until fragrant.

3. Stir in the chickpeas, diced tomatoes, and vegetable broth. Bring to a simmer.

4. Add the cauliflower florets, zucchini, and frozen peas. Simmer for 15•20 minutes, until the vegetables are tender.

5. Remove from heat and stir in the chopped cilantro. Season with salt and pepper to taste.

6. Serve the vegetable curry warm, over steamed brown rice or quinoa if desired.

This curry is diabetes•friendly as it is high in fiber, protein, and complex carbs, while being low in saturated fat and added sugars. The variety of vegetables provide important vitamins, minerals, and antioxidants.

What is the total cooking time, including prep time?

Prep Time : _________________

Cook Time : _________________

Servings : _________________

Ingredients:

- 1 tbsp olive oil
- 1 onion, diced
- 3 cloves garlic, minced
- 1 tbsp grated fresh ginger
- 2 tsp curry powder
- 1 tsp ground cumin
- 1/2 tsp ground coriander
- 1/4 tsp cayenne pepper (optional)
- 1 (15 oz) can chickpeas, rinsed and drained
- 1 (14 oz) can diced tomatoes
- 1 cup low•sodium vegetable broth
- 1 medium cauliflower, cut into florets
- 1 medium zucchini, diced
- 1 cup frozen peas
- 1/4 cup chopped fresh cilantro
- Salt and pepper to taste

Is the recipe easy to follow?

91. Vegetable Curry with Chickpeas

What are the critical points in the recipe (e.g., temperature control, timing)?

What is the total cooking time, including prep time?

Prep Time : _______________

Cook Time : _______________

Servings : _______________

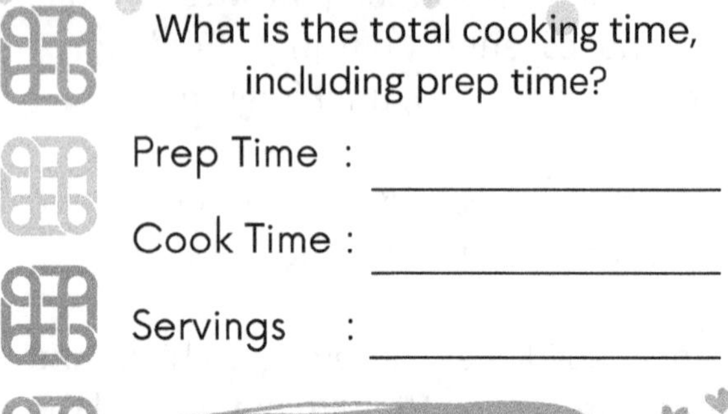

Ingredients:

• 3 medium zucchinis, spiralized or julienned into noodles
• 1/2 cup packed fresh basil leaves
• 2 tbsp pine nuts
• 2 tbsp grated Parmesan cheese
• 1 clove garlic, minced
• 2 tbsp olive oil
• 1 tbsp lemon juice
• Salt and pepper to taste

Is the recipe easy to follow?

92. Zucchini Noodles with Pesto

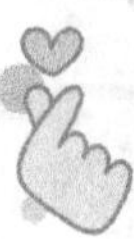

Procedure:

1. In a food processor or blender, combine the basil, pine nuts, Parmesan, and garlic. Pulse until finely chopped.

2. With the motor running, slowly drizzle in the olive oil and lemon juice. Process until a smooth pesto forms. Season with salt and pepper to taste.

3. In a large skillet or sauté pan, bring 1•2 inches of water to a simmer over medium heat. Add the zucchini noodles and cook for 2•3 minutes, just until tender but still crisp. Drain the noodles and pat dry with paper towels.

4. In a large bowl, toss the cooked zucchini noodles with the prepared pesto until evenly coated.

5. Serve the zucchini noodles with pesto immediately, garnished with extra Parmesan cheese if desired.

This dish is diabetes•friendly as it is low in carbs, high in fiber, and contains healthy fats from the olive oil and pine nuts. The zucchini noodles provide a low•calorie alternative to traditional pasta. The pesto adds flavor without a lot of added sugars or sodium.

For seniors over 50 with diabetes, this recipe is a great option as it is easy to prepare, nutrient•dense, and gentle on the digestive system. Enjoy!

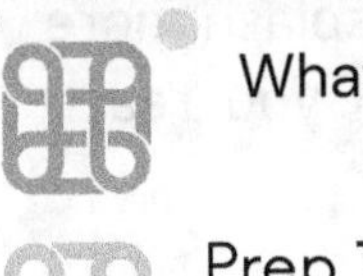

What is the total cooking time, including prep time?

Prep Time   : _________________

Cook Time : _________________

Servings   : _________________

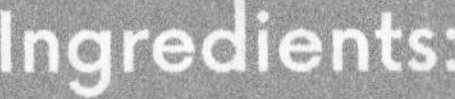
Ingredients:

- 4 large portobello mushroom caps, stems removed and chopped
- 1 tbsp olive oil
- 1/2 cup diced onion
- 2 cloves garlic, minced
- 1 cup baby spinach, chopped
- 1/2 cup diced tomatoes
- 2 tbsp grated Parmesan cheese
- 2 tbsp panko breadcrumbs
- 1 tsp dried oregano
- 1/4 tsp red pepper flakes (optional)
- Salt and pepper to taste
- 1/2 cup shredded part•skim mozzarella cheese

Is the recipe easy to follow?

93. Stuffed Portobello Mushrooms

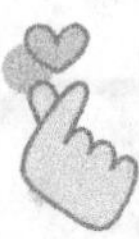
Procedure:

1. Preheat oven to 400°F. Lightly grease a baking sheet.

2. Gently scoop out and chop the mushroom stems, being careful not to tear the caps. Set the caps aside.

3. In a skillet, heat the olive oil over medium heat. Add the chopped mushroom stems, onion, and garlic. Sauté for 3•4 minutes until softened.

4. Stir in the spinach, tomatoes, Parmesan, panko, oregano, and red pepper flakes (if using). Season with salt and pepper.

5. Arrange the mushroom caps on the prepared baking sheet, gill•side up. Spoon the filling evenly into the caps.

6. Top each stuffed mushroom with a sprinkle of the shredded mozzarella cheese.

7. Bake for 15•18 minutes, until the mushrooms are tender and the cheese is melted and bubbly.

8. Serve the stuffed portobello mushrooms warm.

This recipe is diabetes•friendly as it is low in carbs, high in fiber, and contains a good source of protein from the cheese. The mushrooms, spinach, and tomatoes provide important vitamins, minerals, and antioxidants. It's a delicious and nutritious option for seniors over 50 with diabetes.

What are the critical points in the recipe (e.g., temperature control, timing)?

What is the total cooking time, including prep time?

Prep Time : _______________

Cook Time : _______________

Servings   : _______________

Ingredients:

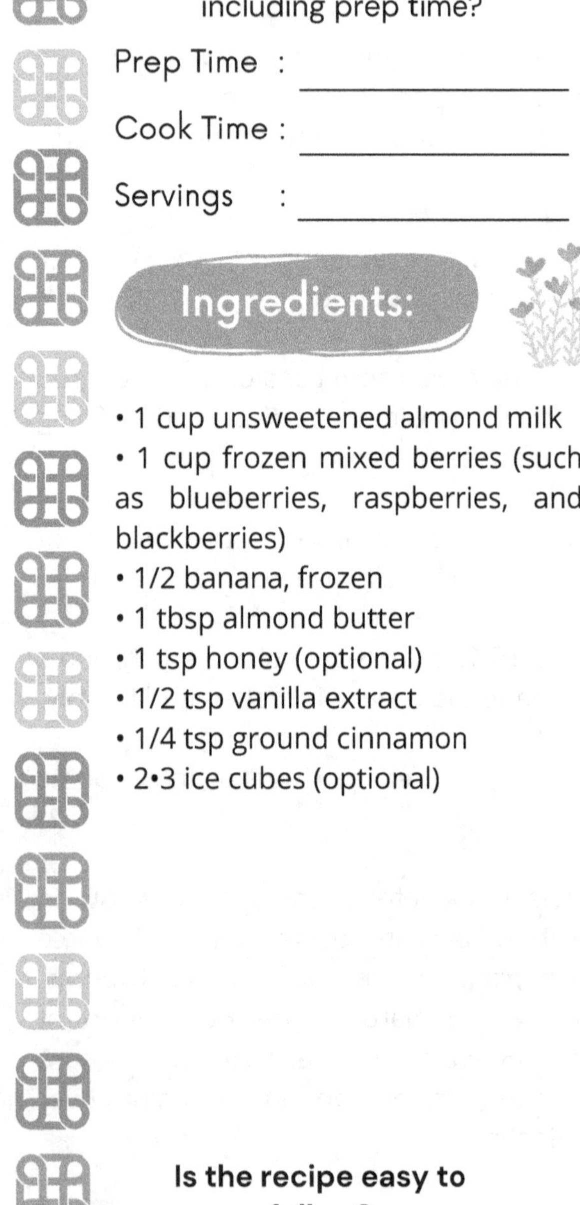

- 1 cup unsweetened almond milk
- 1 cup frozen mixed berries (such as blueberries, raspberries, and blackberries)
- 1/2 banana, frozen
- 1 tbsp almond butter
- 1 tsp honey (optional)
- 1/2 tsp vanilla extract
- 1/4 tsp ground cinnamon
- 2•3 ice cubes (optional)

Is the recipe easy to follow?

☺   ☹

94. Almond Milk Smoothie with Berries

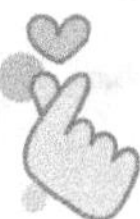

Procedure:

1. Add all the ingredients to a high•powered blender. Blend on high speed until smooth and creamy, about 1•2 minutes.

2. If the smoothie is too thick, add a splash more almond milk and blend again until you reach your desired consistency.

3. Taste and adjust sweetness by adding more honey if desired.

4. Pour the smoothie into a glass and enjoy immediately.

This almond milk smoothie is a great option for a healthy, diabetes•friendly breakfast or snack. Here's why it's a good choice:

- Almond milk is low in carbs and calories, and provides healthy fats and calcium.
- Berries are high in fiber, vitamins, and antioxidants, while being low in sugar.
- Banana adds natural sweetness and creaminess.
- Almond butter provides protein, fiber, and healthy fats to help keep you full.
- Cinnamon may help regulate blood sugar levels.

The combination of nutrients in this smoothie makes it a nutritious and satisfying option for seniors with diabetes. Feel free to adjust the ingredients to your taste preferences. Enjoy!

What are the critical points in the recipe (e.g., temperature control, timing)?

What is the total cooking time, including prep time?

Prep Time : _______________

Cook Time : _______________

Servings   : _______________

• 1 cup unsweetened coconut yogurt
• 1 cup mixed fresh berries (such as blueberries, raspberries, blackberries)
• 1/2 cup diced mango or pineapple
• 1 tbsp unsweetened shredded coconut
• 1 tsp honey (optional)
• 1/4 tsp ground cinnamon

Is the recipe easy to follow?

95. *Coconut Yogurt with Fresh Fruit*

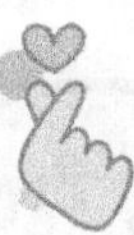

1. In a medium bowl, spoon the coconut yogurt into the bottom.

2. Top the yogurt with the mixed fresh berries and diced mango or pineapple.

3. Sprinkle the unsweetened shredded coconut over the fruit.

4. If desired, drizzle the honey over the top. Sprinkle with the ground cinnamon.

5. Serve chilled or at room temperature.

This coconut yogurt with fresh fruit is a great option for seniors with diabetes for a few reasons:

• Coconut yogurt is high in healthy fats and low in carbs, making it a diabetes•friendly choice.
• The fresh fruits provide fiber, vitamins, and natural sweetness without added sugars.
• Cinnamon may help regulate blood sugar levels.
• The dish is light, refreshing, and easy to digest.

The combination of the creamy coconut yogurt, juicy fresh fruit, and warm spices creates a delicious and nutritious snack or light dessert. Feel free to adjust the fruit selection based on personal preferences or what's in season.

Enjoy this simple yet satisfying coconut yogurt parfait as part of a balanced diabetic diet for seniors over 50.

What is the total cooking time,
including prep time?

Prep Time : _______________

Cook Time : _______________

Servings   : _______________

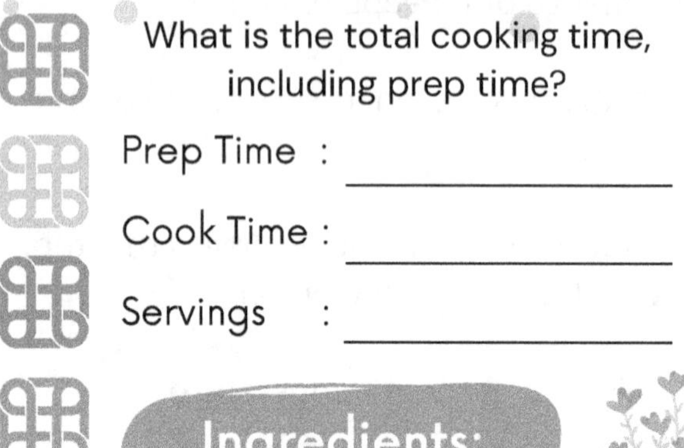

Ingredients:

• 1 cup unsweetened almond milk
• 1/4 cup chia seeds
• 1 tbsp maple syrup (or 1•2 tsp honey)
• 1 tsp vanilla extract
• 1/4 tsp ground cinnamon
• 1/4 cup fresh berries (such as blueberries, raspberries, or chopped strawberries)
• 2 tbsp unsweetened shredded coconut (optional)

Is the recipe easy to follow?

96. Dairy•Free Chia Pudding

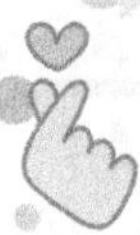

Procedure:

1. In a medium bowl, whisk together the almond milk, chia seeds, maple syrup (or honey), vanilla, and cinnamon until well combined.

2. Cover the bowl and refrigerate for at least 4 hours, or overnight, stirring occasionally, until the chia seeds have thickened the mixture into a pudding•like consistency.

3. When ready to serve, divide the chia pudding evenly between 2•3 serving bowls or glasses.

4. Top each serving with the fresh berries and shredded coconut (if using).

5. Serve chilled.

This dairy•free chia pudding is a great option for a diabetic diet for seniors over 50 for a few reasons:

• Chia seeds are high in fiber, protein, and healthy omega•3 fatty acids, which can help regulate blood sugar levels.
• Almond milk is low in carbs and calories compared to dairy milk.
• The natural sweetness comes from the small amount of maple syrup or honey, which are better options than refined sugar.
• The fresh berries provide additional fiber, vitamins, and antioxidants.
• Cinnamon may help improve insulin sensitivity.

This pudding is easy to prepare, nutrient•dense, and gentle on the digestive system • making it an ideal healthy snack or breakfast for seniors with diabetes. Adjust the sweetener to your taste preference.

What is the total cooking time, including prep time?

Prep Time : _______________

Cook Time : _______________

Servings : _______________

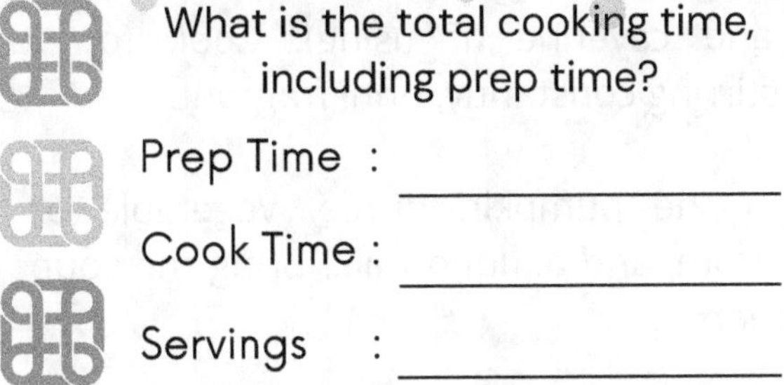

Ingredients:

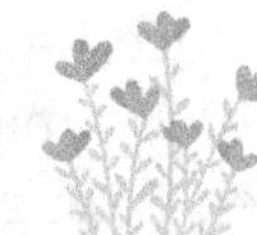

• 1 cup raw cashews, soaked in water for at least 4 hours or overnight
• 2 tbsp lemon juice
• 2 tbsp nutritional yeast
• 1 tsp garlic powder
• 1/2 tsp onion powder
• 1/4 tsp salt
• 2•3 tbsp unsweetened almond milk or water

Vegetables for serving:
• Carrot sticks
• Celery sticks
• Cucumber slices
• Bell pepper strips
• Cherry tomatoes

Is the recipe easy to follow?

97. Cashew Cheese Spread with Vegetables

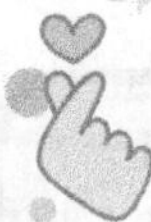

Procedure:

1. Drain and rinse the soaked cashews. Add them to a high•powered blender or food processor.

2. Add the lemon juice, nutritional yeast, garlic powder, onion powder, and salt. Blend until smooth and creamy, adding 2•3 tbsp of almond milk or water as needed to reach your desired consistency.

3. Transfer the cashew cheese spread to a serving bowl.

4. Arrange the assorted vegetable sticks and pieces around the bowl for dipping.

5. Serve immediately or refrigerate until ready to serve.

This cashew cheese spread is a great option for a diabetic diet for seniors over 50 for a few reasons:

• Cashews are high in healthy fats, protein, and fiber, which can help regulate blood sugar levels.
• Nutritional yeast provides a savory, cheese•like flavor without any dairy.
• The vegetables provide fiber, vitamins, and minerals without added sugars or carbs.
• It's a satisfying, nutrient•dense snack or appetizer.

The creamy cashew cheese pairs perfectly with the fresh, crunchy vegetables. Feel free to adjust the seasonings to your taste preferences. This recipe is easy to make and perfect for seniors looking for a diabetes•friendly dip or spread.

What are the critical points in the recipe (e.g., temperature control, timing)?

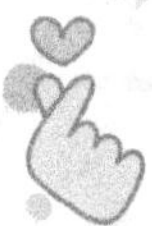

Procedure:

What is the total cooking time, including prep time?

Prep Time : _______________

Cook Time : _______________

Servings   : _______________

Ingredients:

• 1 tbsp olive oil
• 1 onion, diced
• 3 cloves garlic, minced
• 1 tsp ground cumin
• 1/2 tsp ground cinnamon
• 1/4 tsp ground ginger
• 1/4 tsp cayenne pepper (optional)
• 1 (15 oz) can pumpkin puree
• 4 cups low•sodium vegetable or chicken broth
• 1 cup unsweetened almond milk
• 1 tsp maple syrup (optional)
• Salt and pepper to taste
• Chopped fresh parsley or chives for garnish

Is the recipe easy to follow?

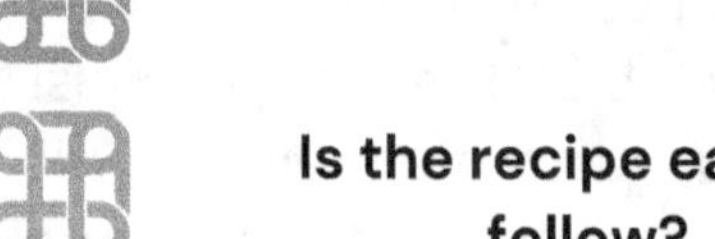
98. Dairy•Free Pumpkin Soup

1. In a large pot or Dutch oven, heat the olive oil over medium heat. Add the diced onion and sauté for 3•4 minutes until translucent.

2. Add the minced garlic, cumin, cinnamon, ginger, and cayenne (if using). Cook for 1 minute, stirring constantly, until fragrant.

3. Stir in the pumpkin puree, vegetable or chicken broth, and almond milk. Bring the soup to a simmer.

4. Reduce heat to low and let the soup simmer for 10•15 minutes, stirring occasionally, until heated through.

5. If desired, stir in the maple syrup to add a touch of sweetness.

6. Season the soup with salt and pepper to taste.

7. Ladle the pumpkin soup into bowls and garnish with chopped fresh parsley or chives.

This dairy•free pumpkin soup is a great option for a diabetic diet for seniors over 50 for a few reasons:

• Pumpkin is low in carbs and high in fiber, vitamins, and antioxidants.
• Almond milk provides creaminess without the dairy.
• The spices like cinnamon and ginger may help regulate blood sugar levels.
• It's a warm, comforting, and nutrient•dense soup.

This soup can be enjoyed as a starter or a light main course. Adjust the amount of maple syrup to your taste preferences. Enjoy!

What is the total cooking time, including prep time?

Prep Time : ______________

Cook Time : ______________

Servings   : ______________

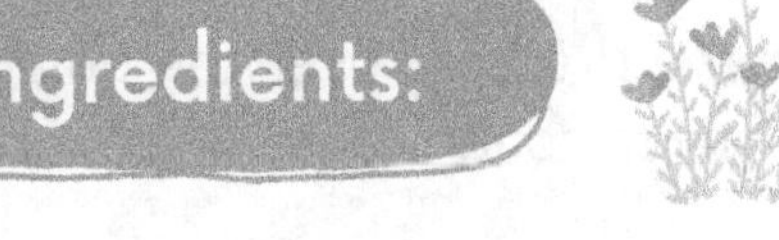
Ingredients:

• 8 oz gluten•free pasta (such as brown rice, quinoa, or chickpea pasta)
• 1 tbsp olive oil
• 1 onion, diced
• 3 cloves garlic, minced
• 1 (28 oz) can crushed tomatoes
• 2 tbsp tomato paste
• 1 tsp dried oregano
• 1/2 tsp dried basil
• 1/4 tsp red pepper flakes (optional)
• Salt and pepper to taste
• 2 tbsp grated Parmesan cheese (optional)
• Chopped fresh basil for garnish

Is the recipe easy to follow?

99. Gluten•Free Pasta with Marinara Sauce

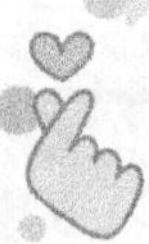
Procedure:

1. Bring a large pot of salted water to a boil. Cook the gluten•free pasta according to package instructions until al dente. Drain and set aside.

2. In a large skillet, heat the olive oil over medium heat. Add the diced onion and sauté for 3•4 minutes until translucent.

3. Add the minced garlic and cook for 1 minute, stirring constantly, until fragrant.

4. Stir in the crushed tomatoes, tomato paste, oregano, dried basil, and red pepper flakes (if using). Season with salt and pepper.

5. Reduce the heat to low and let the marinara sauce simmer for 10•15 minutes, stirring occasionally, until thickened.

6. Add the cooked gluten•free pasta to the sauce and toss to coat evenly.

7. Serve the pasta with marinara sauce warm, topped with a sprinkle of Parmesan cheese (if using) and chopped fresh basil.

This gluten•free pasta dish is a great option for a diabetic diet for seniors over 50 for a few reasons:

• Gluten•free pasta is lower in carbs and higher in fiber compared to traditional wheat pasta.
• The marinara sauce is low in added sugars and high in lycopene from the tomatoes.
• The dish is easy to digest and gentle on the stomach.

Feel free to adjust the amount of red pepper flakes or Parmesan cheese to your taste preferences. Enjoy this diabetes•friendly pasta dish!

What are the critical points in the recipe (e.g., temperature control, timing)?

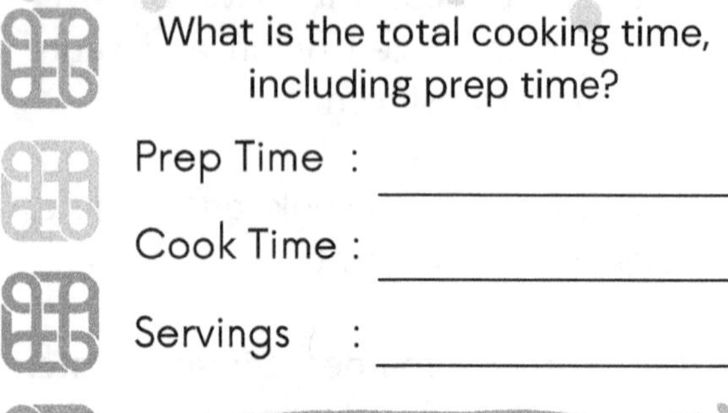

What is the total cooking time, including prep time?

Prep Time : _______________

Cook Time : _______________

Servings : _______________

Ingredients:

• 1 cup uncooked quinoa, rinsed
• 2 cups low•sodium vegetable or chicken broth
• 1 (15 oz) can black beans, rinsed and drained
• 1 avocado, diced
• 1 cup cherry tomatoes, halved
• 1/2 cup diced red onion
• 1/4 cup chopped fresh cilantro
• 2 tbsp olive oil
• 2 tbsp lime juice
• 1 tsp ground cumin
• 1/4 tsp chili powder
• Salt and pepper to taste

Is the recipe easy to follow?

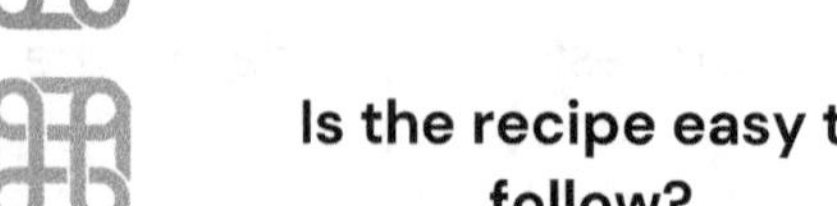

100. Quinoa Salad with Avocado and Black Beans

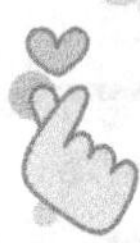

Procedure:

1. In a medium saucepan, combine the quinoa and broth. Bring to a boil, then reduce heat to low, cover and simmer for 15•20 minutes, until quinoa is tender and liquid is absorbed. Fluff with a fork and let cool slightly.

2. In a large bowl, combine the cooked quinoa, black beans, diced avocado, cherry tomatoes, red onion, and chopped cilantro.

3. In a small bowl, whisk together the olive oil, lime juice, cumin, and chili powder.

4. Pour the dressing over the quinoa salad and toss gently to coat.

5. Season the salad with salt and pepper to taste.

6. Serve the quinoa salad chilled or at room temperature.

This quinoa salad is a great option for a healthy, diabetes•friendly meal or side dish. Here's why it's a good choice:

• Quinoa is a gluten•free whole grain that's high in fiber and protein.
• Black beans provide additional fiber, protein, and complex carbs.
• Avocado contributes healthy fats and creaminess.
• The vegetables add vitamins, minerals, and antioxidants.
• The lime juice and spices add flavor without added sugars.

This salad is easy to prepare, nutrient•dense, and filling. It's perfect for seniors over 50 with diabetes who are looking for a tasty, balanced meal. Adjust the ingredients to your taste preferences.

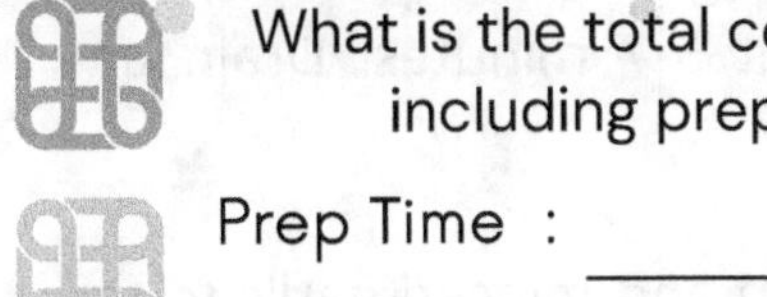

What is the total cooking time, including prep time?

Prep Time : ________________

Cook Time : ________________

Servings   : ________________

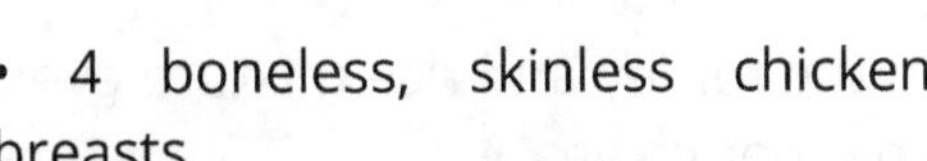
Ingredients:

• 4 boneless, skinless chicken breasts
• 1 tbsp olive oil
• 1 tsp garlic powder
• 1 tsp dried oregano
• Salt and pepper to taste
• 1 cup uncooked quinoa, rinsed
• 2 cups low•sodium chicken or vegetable broth
• 1 cup diced zucchini
• 1 cup diced bell pepper
• 1/2 cup diced onion
• 2 tbsp chopped fresh parsley

Is the recipe easy to follow?

101. Grilled Chicken with Quinoa and Vegetables

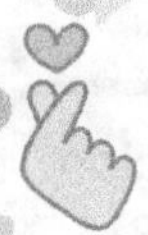
Procedure:

1. Preheat grill or grill pan to medium•high heat.

2. Rub the chicken breasts with the olive oil and season with the garlic powder, oregano, salt, and pepper.

3. Grill the chicken for 5•7 minutes per side, or until cooked through. Transfer to a plate and let rest for 5 minutes before slicing.

4. In a medium saucepan, combine the quinoa and broth. Bring to a boil, then reduce heat to low, cover and simmer for 15•20 minutes, until quinoa is tender and liquid is absorbed.

5. While the quinoa is cooking, sauté the diced zucchini, bell pepper, and onion in a skillet over medium heat for 5•7 minutes, until tender.

6. Fluff the cooked quinoa with a fork and stir in the sautéed vegetables and chopped parsley.

7. Serve the grilled chicken sliced over the quinoa vegetable mixture.

This grilled chicken and quinoa dish is an excellent choice for a diabetic diet for seniors over 50 for several reasons:

• Chicken is a lean protein that is low in fat and carbs.
• Quinoa is a whole grain that is high in fiber, protein, and complex carbs.
• The vegetables provide important vitamins, minerals, and antioxidants.

The combination of the juicy grilled chicken, fluffy quinoa, and fresh vegetables makes for a nutritious and flavorful meal. Feel free to adjust the vegetable selection based on personal preferences. Enjoy!

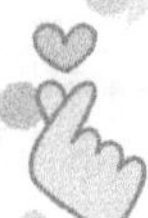

What is the total cooking time, including prep time?

Prep Time : _______________

Cook Time : _______________

Servings : _______________

Ingredients:

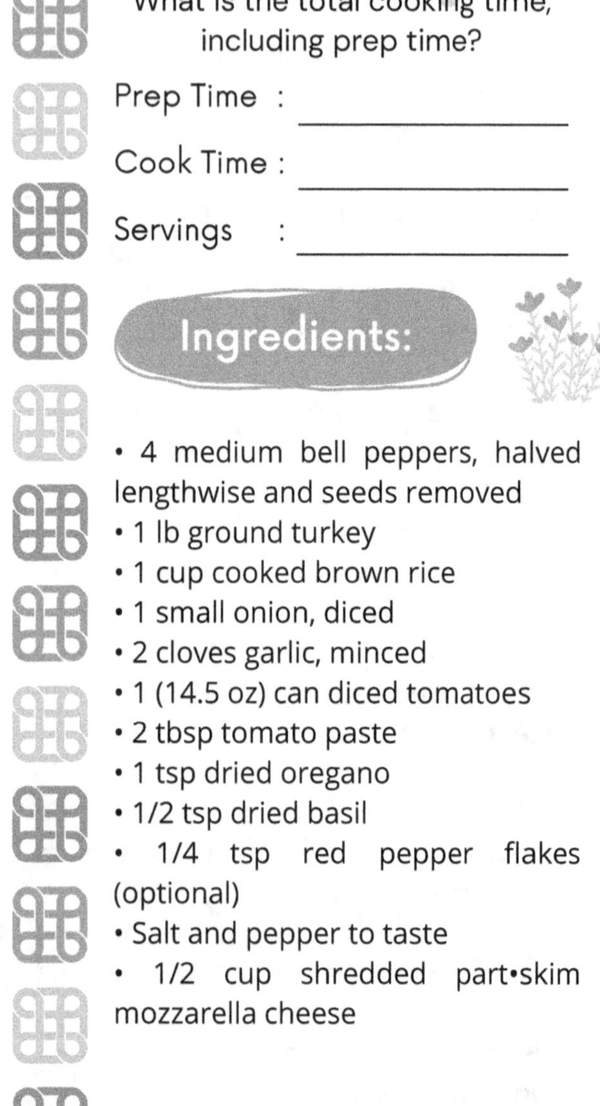

• 4 medium bell peppers, halved lengthwise and seeds removed
• 1 lb ground turkey
• 1 cup cooked brown rice
• 1 small onion, diced
• 2 cloves garlic, minced
• 1 (14.5 oz) can diced tomatoes
• 2 tbsp tomato paste
• 1 tsp dried oregano
• 1/2 tsp dried basil
• 1/4 tsp red pepper flakes (optional)
• Salt and pepper to taste
• 1/2 cup shredded part•skim mozzarella cheese

Is the recipe easy to follow?

🙂 🙁

102. Stuffed Bell Peppers with Ground Turkey and Rice

1. Preheat oven to 375°F. Arrange the bell pepper halves in a baking dish.

2. In a large skillet over medium heat, cook the ground turkey, breaking it up as it cooks, until no longer pink, about 5•7 minutes. Drain any excess fat.

3. Add the diced onion and minced garlic to the skillet. Cook for 2•3 minutes until the onion is translucent.

4. Stir in the cooked brown rice, diced tomatoes, tomato paste, oregano, basil, and red pepper flakes (if using). Season with salt and pepper.

5. Spoon the turkey and rice mixture evenly into the bell pepper halves.

6. Top each stuffed pepper with a sprinkle of the shredded mozzarella cheese.

7. Cover the baking dish with foil and bake for 25•30 minutes, until the peppers are tender.

8. Remove the foil and bake for an additional 5 minutes, until the cheese is melted and lightly browned. Serve the stuffed bell peppers warm.

This stuffed bell pepper dish is a great option for a diabetic diet for seniors over 50 for several reasons:

• Bell peppers are low in carbs and high in fiber, vitamins, and antioxidants.
• Ground turkey is a lean protein that is low in fat and carbs.
• Brown rice provides complex carbs and additional fiber.
• The dish is well•balanced, satisfying, and easy to digest.

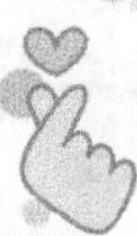

What are the critical points in the recipe (e.g., temperature control, timing)?

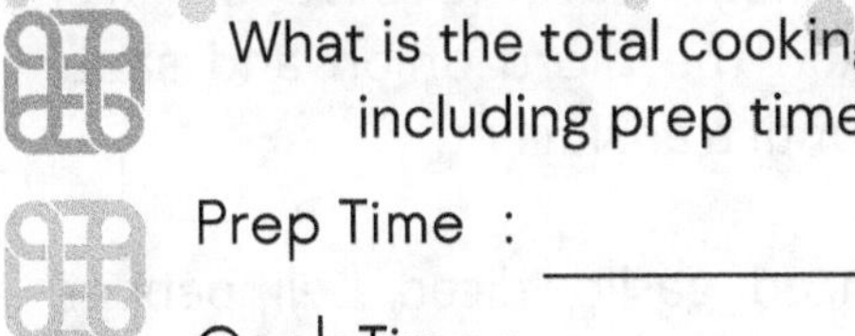

What is the total cooking time, including prep time?

Prep Time : _______________

Cook Time : _______________

Servings   : _______________

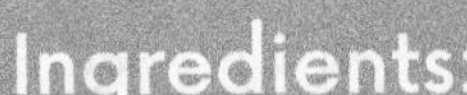
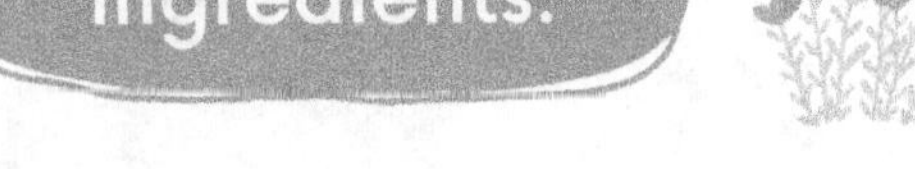

Ingredients:

- 2 tbsp coconut oil or avocado oil
- 1 cup sliced mushrooms
- 1 cup broccoli florets
- 1 cup sliced bell peppers
- 1 cup shredded cabbage
- 1 cup snow peas or snap peas
- 3 cloves garlic, minced
- 1 tbsp grated fresh ginger
- 2 tbsp gluten•free tamari or coconut aminos
- 1 tsp sesame oil
- 1/4 tsp red pepper flakes (optional)
- Salt and pepper to taste
- 2 cups cooked quinoa or brown rice (for serving)

Is the recipe easy to follow?

103. Gluten•Free Veggie Stir•Fry

Procedure:

1. In a large wok or skillet, heat the coconut or avocado oil over medium•high heat.

2. Add the sliced mushrooms, broccoli florets, bell pepper slices, shredded cabbage, and snow/snap peas. Stir•fry for 5•7 minutes, until the vegetables are crisp•tender.

3. Push the vegetables to the side of the pan. Add the minced garlic and grated ginger to the center of the pan. Cook for 1 minute, stirring constantly, until fragrant.

4. Stir the garlic and ginger into the vegetables. Add the gluten•free tamari or coconut aminos, sesame oil, and red pepper flakes (if using). Toss everything together and season with salt and pepper to taste.

5. Serve the stir•fried vegetables immediately, over a bed of cooked quinoa or brown rice.

This gluten•free veggie stir•fry is an excellent choice for a diabetic diet for seniors over 50 for several reasons:

- It's low in carbs and high in fiber, vitamins, and minerals from the variety of vegetables.
- The quinoa or brown rice provides complex carbs and additional fiber.
- The dish is easy to digest and gentle on the stomach.
- It's a flavorful, satisfying, and diabetes•friendly meal.

The combination of the crisp•tender veggies, savory sauce, and nutty whole grains makes this stir•fry a nutritious and delicious option. Feel free to adjust the vegetable selection based on personal preferences. Enjoy!

What are the critical points in the recipe (e.g., temperature control, timing)?

What is the total cooking time, including prep time?

Prep Time : _________________

Cook Time : _________________

Servings : _________________

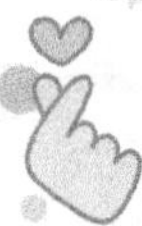

Ingredients:

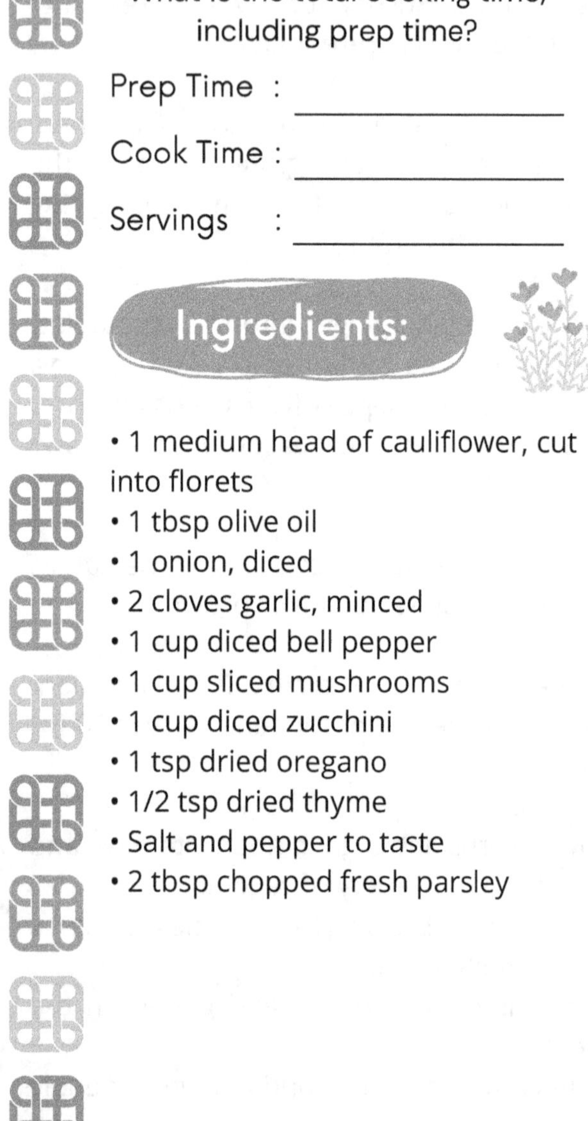

• 1 medium head of cauliflower, cut into florets
• 1 tbsp olive oil
• 1 onion, diced
• 2 cloves garlic, minced
• 1 cup diced bell pepper
• 1 cup sliced mushrooms
• 1 cup diced zucchini
• 1 tsp dried oregano
• 1/2 tsp dried thyme
• Salt and pepper to taste
• 2 tbsp chopped fresh parsley

Is the recipe easy to follow?

104. Cauliflower Rice with Sautéed Vegetables

1. In a food processor, pulse the cauliflower florets until they resemble rice•sized grains. Set aside.

2. In a large skillet, heat the olive oil over medium heat. Add the diced onion and sauté for 3•4 minutes until translucent.

3. Add the minced garlic, diced bell pepper, sliced mushrooms, and diced zucchini. Sauté for 5•7 minutes, until the vegetables are tender.

4. Stir in the riced cauliflower, dried oregano, and dried thyme. Season with salt and pepper to taste.

5. Cook the cauliflower rice and vegetables for 5•7 minutes, stirring occasionally, until the cauliflower is tender.

6. Remove from heat and stir in the chopped fresh parsley.

7. Serve the cauliflower rice and sautéed vegetables warm.

This cauliflower rice dish is an excellent option for a diabetic diet for seniors over 50 for several reasons:

• Cauliflower is low in carbs and calories, but high in fiber, vitamins, and minerals.
• The sautéed vegetables provide additional nutrients, antioxidants, and fiber.
• The dish is easy to digest and gentle on the stomach.
• It's a flavorful, satisfying, and diabetes•friendly meal or side dish.

What is the total cooking time, including prep time?

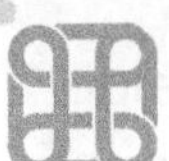
Prep Time : _______________

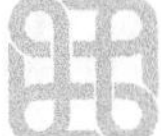
Cook Time : _______________

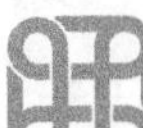
Servings   : _______________

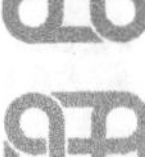

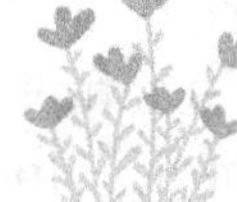

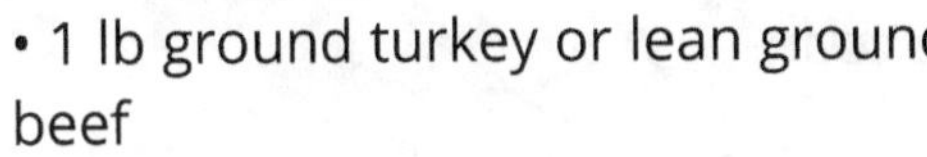
Ingredients:

For the Meatballs:
• 1 lb ground turkey or lean ground beef
• 1/2 cup grated Parmesan cheese
• 1 egg
• 1/4 cup almond flour
• 2 cloves garlic, minced
• 1 tsp dried oregano
• 1/2 tsp salt
• 1/4 tsp black pepper

For the Zucchini Noodles:
• 3 medium zucchinis, spiralized or julienned into noodles
• 1 tbsp olive oil
• 2 cloves garlic, minced
• 1 (24 oz) jar low•sugar marinara sauce
• 1/4 cup chopped fresh basil

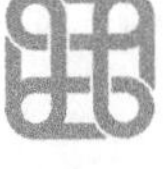

Is the recipe easy to follow?

105. Zucchini Noodles with Meatballs

Procedure:

1. Preheat oven to 400°F. Line a baking sheet with parchment paper.

2. In a large bowl, combine all the meatball ingredients and mix well. Roll the mixture into 1•inch meatballs and place them on the prepared baking sheet.

3. Bake the meatballs for 18•20 minutes, until cooked through.

4. While the meatballs are baking, heat the olive oil in a large skillet over medium heat. Add the minced garlic and cook for 1 minute until fragrant.

5. Add the spiralized or julienned zucchini noodles to the skillet. Sauté for 3•5 minutes, until the zucchini is tender but still has some bite.

6. Pour the low•sugar marinara sauce over the zucchini noodles and toss to coat.

7. Add the cooked meatballs to the skillet and gently toss to combine.

8. Serve the zucchini noodles and meatballs warm, garnished with the chopped fresh basil.

This zucchini noodle and meatball dish is a great option for a diabetic diet for seniors over 50 for several reasons:

• Zucchini noodles are low in carbs and calories, but high in fiber and nutrients.
• Ground turkey or beef provides lean protein without too much saturated fat.
• The low•sugar marinara sauce keeps the carb content in check.
• It's a satisfying, well•balanced meal that's easy to digest.

What are the critical points in the recipe (e.g., temperature control, timing)?

What is the total cooking time, including prep time?

Prep Time : _______________

Cook Time : _______________

Servings   : _______________

Ingredients:

For the Grilled Chicken:
• 4 boneless, skinless chicken breasts
• 2 tbsp olive oil
• 1 tsp garlic powder
• 1 tsp dried oregano
• Salt and pepper to taste

For the Side Salad:
• 6 cups mixed greens (such as spinach, arugula, and romaine)
• 1 cup cherry tomatoes, halved
• 1/2 cucumber, sliced
• 1/4 red onion, thinly sliced
• 2 tbsp olive oil
• 1 tbsp balsamic vinegar
• 1 tsp Dijon mustard
• 1 tsp honey
• Salt and pepper to taste

Is the recipe easy to follow?

🙂   ☹️

106. Grilled Chicken with a Side Salad

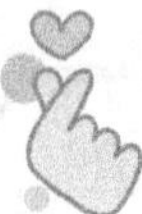

Procedure:

For the Grilled Chicken:
1. Preheat grill or grill pan to medium•high heat.
2. Rub the chicken breasts all over with the olive oil and season with the garlic powder, oregano, salt, and pepper.
3. Grill the chicken for 5•7 minutes per side, until cooked through. Transfer to a plate and let rest for 5 minutes before slicing.

For the Side Salad:
1. In a large bowl, combine the mixed greens, cherry tomatoes, cucumber slices, and red onion.
2. In a small bowl, whisk together the olive oil, balsamic vinegar, Dijon mustard, and honey. Season with salt and pepper.
3. Drizzle the dressing over the salad and toss gently to coat.

To Serve:
1. Divide the grilled chicken slices and side salad evenly between 4 plates.

This grilled chicken with a side salad is an excellent choice for a diabetic diet for seniors over 50 for several reasons:

• Chicken is a lean protein that is low in fat and carbs.
• The mixed greens, tomatoes, cucumber, and onion provide fiber, vitamins, and antioxidants.
• The simple olive oil and balsamic vinegar dressing is low in added sugars.
• It's a well•balanced, nutrient•dense meal that's easy to digest.

The combination of the juicy grilled chicken and the fresh, crunchy salad makes for a satisfying and diabetes•friendly dish. Feel free to adjust the salad ingredients based on personal preferences. Enjoy!

What are the critical points in the recipe (e.g., temperature control, timing)?

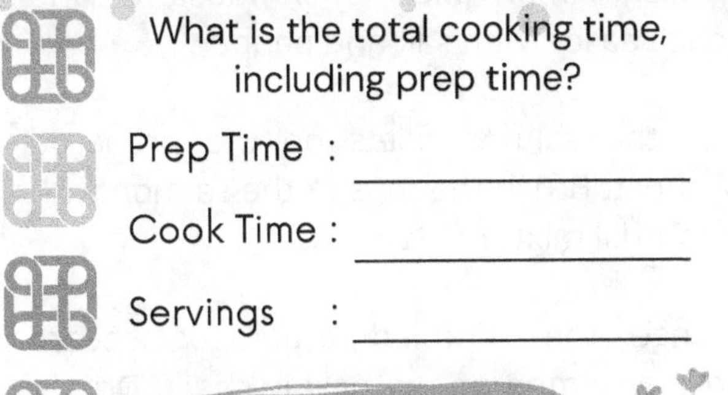

What is the total cooking time, including prep time?

Prep Time : _______________

Cook Time : _______________

Servings   : _______________

Ingredients:

- 2 medium eggplants, sliced lengthwise into 1/4•inch thick slices
- 1 tbsp olive oil
- 1 onion, diced
- 3 cloves garlic, minced
- 1 (28 oz) can crushed tomatoes
- 2 tbsp tomato paste
- 1 tsp dried oregano
- 1/2 tsp dried basil
- Salt and pepper to taste
- 1 cup part•skim ricotta cheese
- 1 egg
- 1/4 cup grated Parmesan cheese
- 2 cups shredded part•skim mozzarella cheese

Is the recipe easy to follow?

107. Eggplant Lasagna

1. Preheat oven to 375°F. Lightly grease a 9x13 inch baking dish.

2. Arrange the eggplant slices in a single layer on a baking sheet. Brush both sides lightly with olive oil. Bake for 15•20 minutes, flipping halfway, until eggplant is tender.

3. In a large skillet, heat 1 tbsp olive oil over medium heat. Add the diced onion and sauté for 3•4 minutes until translucent. Add the minced garlic and cook for 1 minute more.

4. Stir in the crushed tomatoes, tomato paste, oregano, and basil. Season with salt and pepper. Simmer the sauce for 10•15 minutes, stirring occasionally, until thickened.

5. In a medium bowl, mix together the ricotta cheese, egg, and 2 tbsp of the Parmesan cheese.

6. Spread 1 cup of the tomato sauce in the bottom of the prepared baking dish. Layer half of the roasted eggplant slices over the sauce. Spread the ricotta mixture evenly over the eggplant. Top with 1 cup of the mozzarella cheese.

7. Add another layer of eggplant slices, then the remaining tomato sauce. Top with the remaining mozzarella and Parmesan cheeses.

8. Bake for 30•35 minutes, until the cheese is melted and bubbly. Let stand for 10 minutes before serving.

Enjoy this delicious and diabetes•friendly eggplant lasagna!

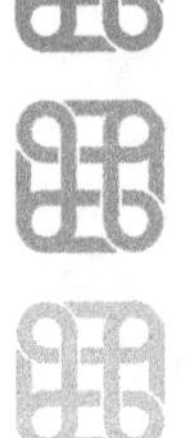
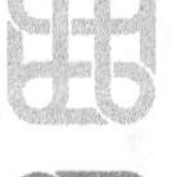
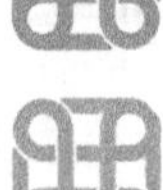

What is the total cooking time, including prep time?

Prep Time : ___________________

Cook Time : ___________________

Servings   : ___________________

Ingredients:

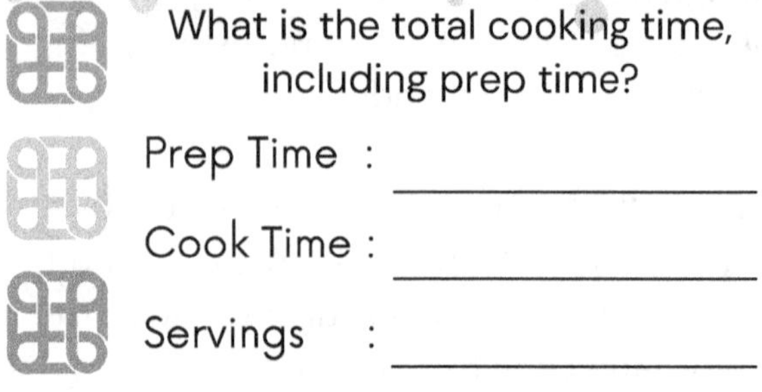

- 4 (6 oz) salmon fillets
- 1 tbsp olive oil
- 1 tsp lemon zest
- 1 tbsp lemon juice
- 1 tsp Dijon mustard
- 1 tsp dried dill
- Salt and pepper to taste
- 1 lb asparagus spears, trimmed
- 1 tbsp unsalted butter, melted

Is the recipe easy to follow?

108. Baked Salmon with Asparagus

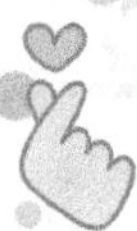

Procedure:

1. Preheat oven to 400°F. Line a baking sheet with parchment paper.

2. In a small bowl, whisk together the olive oil, lemon zest, lemon juice, Dijon mustard, and dried dill. Season with salt and pepper.

3. Place the salmon fillets on the prepared baking sheet. Brush the tops of the salmon with the lemon•dill mixture.

4. Arrange the trimmed asparagus spears around the salmon on the baking sheet. Drizzle the melted butter over the asparagus.

5. Bake for 12•15 minutes, until the salmon is opaque and flakes easily with a fork, and the asparagus is tender•crisp.

6. Serve the baked salmon and asparagus immediately.

This baked salmon and asparagus dish is an excellent choice for a diabetic diet for seniors over 50 for several reasons:

- Salmon is a fatty fish that is high in heart•healthy omega•3 fatty acids.
- Asparagus is low in carbs and high in fiber, vitamins, and antioxidants.
- The lemon•dill sauce provides flavor without added sugars.
- It's a well•balanced, nutrient•dense meal that's easy to digest.

The combination of the tender, flavorful salmon and the crisp•tender asparagus makes for a delicious and diabetes•friendly dish. The simple preparation also makes it easy to prepare for seniors.

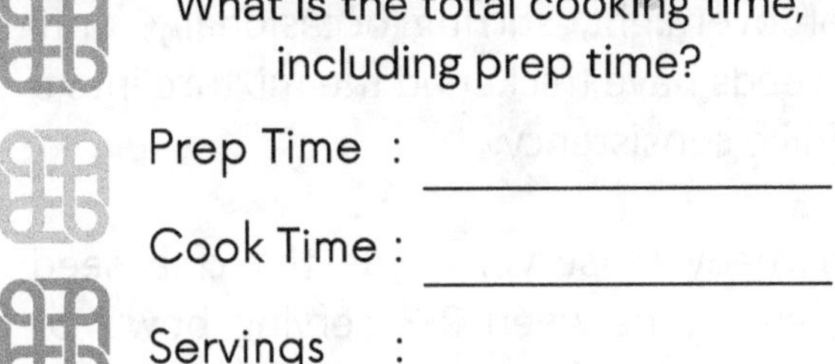

What is the total cooking time, including prep time?

Prep Time : ________________

Cook Time : ________________

Servings   : ________________

Ingredients:

• 1 lb large shrimp, peeled and deveined
• 3 tbsp olive oil
• 4 cloves garlic, minced
• 1/4 cup dry white wine or low•sodium chicken broth
• 2 tbsp fresh lemon juice
• 2 tbsp unsalted butter
• 1/4 cup chopped fresh parsley
• Salt and pepper to taste
• 3 medium zucchinis, spiralized or julienned into noodles

Is the recipe easy to follow?

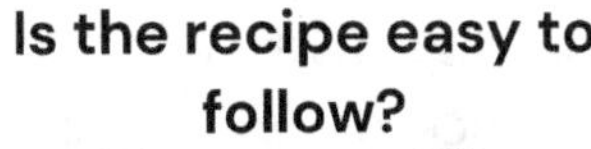

109. Shrimp Scampi with Zucchini Noodles

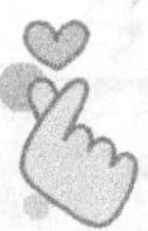

Procedure:

1. In a large skillet, heat 2 tbsp of the olive oil over medium•high heat. Add the shrimp and cook for 2•3 minutes per side, until opaque and cooked through. Transfer the shrimp to a plate and set aside.

2. In the same skillet, heat the remaining 1 tbsp of olive oil over medium heat. Add the minced garlic and cook for 1 minute, until fragrant.

3. Pour in the white wine (or chicken broth) and lemon juice. Bring the mixture to a simmer and cook for 2•3 minutes, until slightly reduced.

4. Reduce the heat to low and stir in the butter until melted and the sauce is creamy.

5. Add the cooked shrimp back to the skillet and toss to coat in the garlic•lemon sauce. Stir in the chopped parsley.

6. In a separate skillet, heat a small amount of olive oil over medium•high heat. Add the spiralized or julienned zucchini noodles and sauté for 3•5 minutes, until tender but still crisp.

7. Divide the zucchini noodles between plates and top with the shrimp scampi.

8. Season with salt and pepper to taste.

This shrimp scampi with zucchini noodles is a great option for a diabetic diet for several reasons:

• Shrimp is a lean protein that is low In carbs and calories.
• Zucchini noodles are a low•carb, high•fiber alternative to traditional pasta.
• The garlic•lemon sauce provides flavor without added sugars.

What is the total cooking time, including prep time?

Prep Time : _________________

Cook Time : _________________

Servings   : _________________

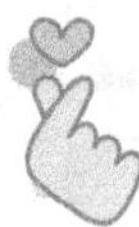

Procedure:

Ingredients:

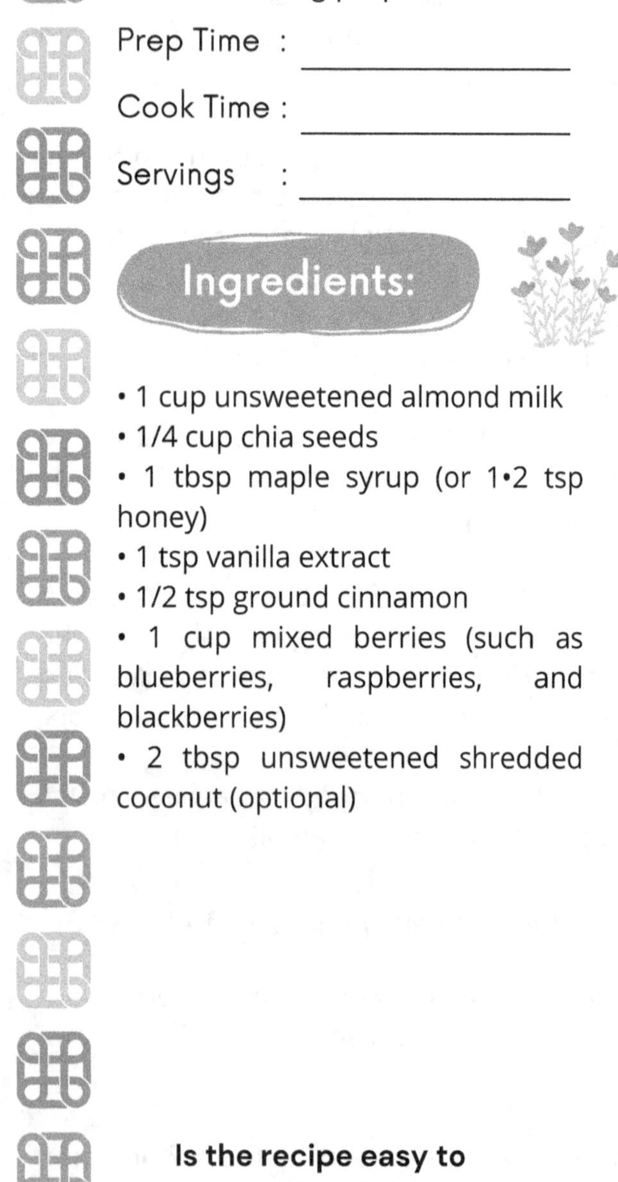

- 1 cup unsweetened almond milk
- 1/4 cup chia seeds
- 1 tbsp maple syrup (or 1•2 tsp honey)
- 1 tsp vanilla extract
- 1/2 tsp ground cinnamon
- 1 cup mixed berries (such as blueberries, raspberries, and blackberries)
- 2 tbsp unsweetened shredded coconut (optional)

Is the recipe easy to follow?

110. Chia Seed Pudding with Berries

1. In a medium bowl, whisk together the almond milk, chia seeds, maple syrup (or honey), vanilla, and cinnamon until well combined.

2. Cover the bowl and refrigerate for at least 4 hours, or overnight, stirring occasionally, until the chia seeds have thickened the mixture into a pudding•like consistency.

3. When ready to serve, divide the chia seed pudding evenly between 2•3 serving bowls or glasses.

4. Top each serving with the mixed berries and shredded coconut (if using).

5. Serve chilled.

This chia seed pudding is a great option for a diabetic diet for seniors over 50 for several reasons:

- Chia seeds are high in fiber, protein, and healthy omega•3 fatty acids, which can help regulate blood sugar levels.
- Almond milk is low in carbs and calories compared to dairy milk.
- The natural sweetness comes from a small amount of maple syrup or honey, which are better options than refined sugar.
- The fresh berries provide additional fiber, vitamins, and antioxidants.
- Cinnamon may help improve insulin sensitivity.

This pudding is easy to prepare, nutrient•dense, and gentle on the digestive system • making it an ideal healthy snack or breakfast for seniors with diabetes. Adjust the sweetener to your taste preference.

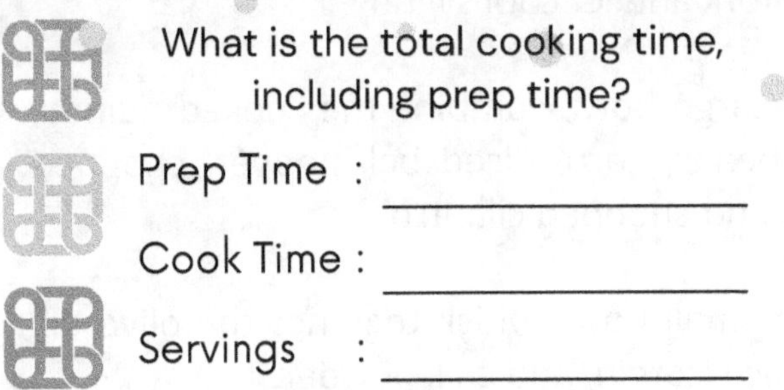

What is the total cooking time, including prep time?

Prep Time : _______________

Cook Time : _______________

Servings   : _______________

Ingredients:

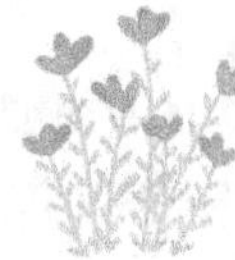

- 1 tbsp olive oil
- 1 onion, diced
- 3 carrots, peeled and diced
- 3 celery stalks, diced
- 3 cloves garlic, minced
- 1 tsp ground cumin
- 1 tsp dried oregano
- 1/4 tsp red pepper flakes (optional)
- 1 cup brown or green lentils, rinsed
- 6 cups low•sodium vegetable or chicken broth
- 1 (14.5 oz) can diced tomatoes
- 2 cups chopped kale or spinach
- Salt and pepper to taste
- Chopped fresh parsley for garnish

Is the recipe easy to follow?

111. Lentil Soup with Vegetables

Procedure:

1. In a large pot or Dutch oven, heat the olive oil over medium heat. Add the diced onion, carrots, and celery. Sauté for 5•7 minutes until the vegetables start to soften.

2. Add the minced garlic, cumin, oregano, and red pepper flakes (if using). Cook for 1 minute, stirring constantly, until fragrant.

3. Stir in the rinsed lentils, broth, and diced tomatoes. Bring the soup to a boil.

4. Reduce the heat to low, cover, and simmer for 20•25 minutes, until the lentils are tender.

5. Stir in the chopped kale or spinach and cook for 5 more minutes, until the greens are wilted.

6. Season the soup with salt and pepper to taste.

7. Ladle the lentil soup into bowls and garnish with chopped fresh parsley.

This lentil soup is a great option for a healthy, diabetes•friendly meal. Here's why:

- Lentils are high in fiber, protein, and complex carbs, which help regulate blood sugar levels.
- The variety of vegetables provide important vitamins, minerals, and antioxidants.
- It's a hearty, satisfying soup that's easy to digest.
- The recipe is simple to prepare and can be easily customized.

For seniors over 50 with diabetes, this lentil soup makes for a nutritious and comforting meal. Adjust the spices and vegetable selection to your taste preferences. Enjoy!

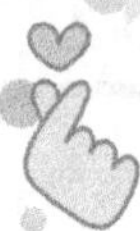

What is the total cooking time, including prep time?

Prep Time : _______________

Cook Time : _______________

Servings : _______________

Ingredients:

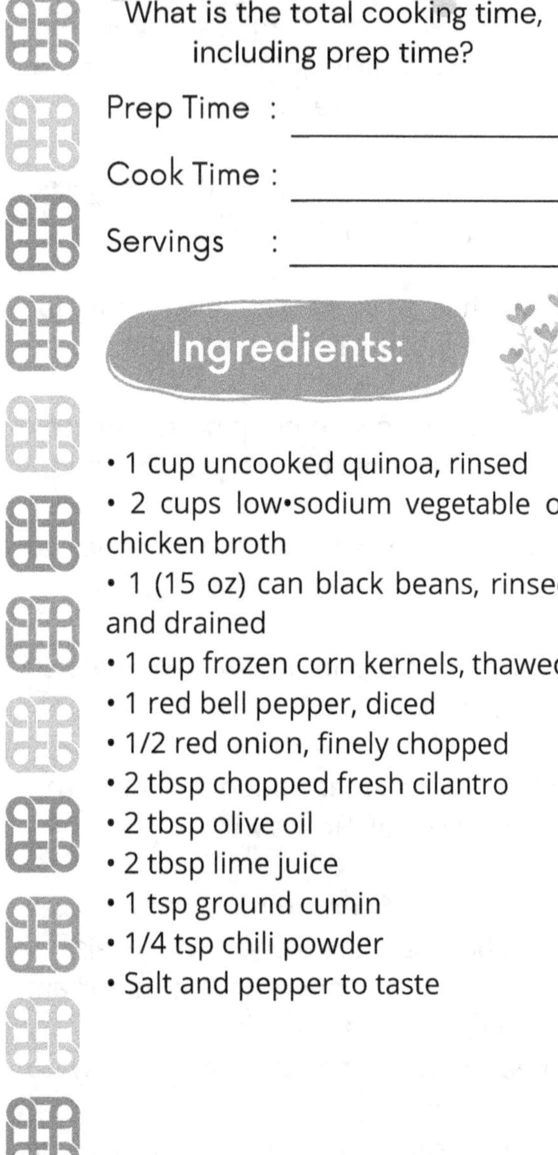

- 1 cup uncooked quinoa, rinsed
- 2 cups low•sodium vegetable or chicken broth
- 1 (15 oz) can black beans, rinsed and drained
- 1 cup frozen corn kernels, thawed
- 1 red bell pepper, diced
- 1/2 red onion, finely chopped
- 2 tbsp chopped fresh cilantro
- 2 tbsp olive oil
- 2 tbsp lime juice
- 1 tsp ground cumin
- 1/4 tsp chili powder
- Salt and pepper to taste

Is the recipe easy to follow?

112. Quinoa Salad with Black Beans and Corn

1. In a medium saucepan, combine the quinoa and broth. Bring to a boil, then reduce heat to low, cover and simmer for 15•20 minutes, until quinoa is tender and liquid is absorbed. Fluff with a fork and let cool slightly.

2. In a large bowl, combine the cooked quinoa, black beans, corn, diced bell pepper, chopped onion, and chopped cilantro.

3. In a small bowl, whisk together the olive oil, lime juice, cumin, and chili powder.

4. Pour the dressing over the quinoa salad and toss gently to coat.

5. Season the salad with salt and pepper to taste.

6. Serve the quinoa salad chilled or at room temperature.

This quinoa salad is a great option for a diabetic diet for seniors over 50 for several reasons:

- Quinoa is a gluten•free whole grain that's high in fiber and protein.
- Black beans provide additional fiber, protein, and complex carbs.
- The vegetables add important vitamins, minerals, and antioxidants.
- The lime juice and spices add flavor without added sugars.

The combination of the nutrient•dense ingredients makes this salad a satisfying and diabetes•friendly meal or side dish. It's easy to prepare and can be enjoyed chilled or at room temperature. Adjust the ingredients to your taste preferences.

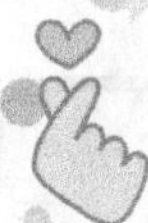

What are the critical points in the recipe (e.g., temperature control, timing)?

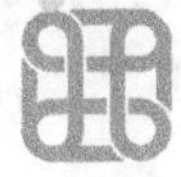
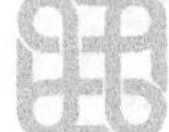

What is the total cooking time, including prep time?

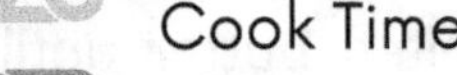

Prep Time : _______________

Cook Time : _______________

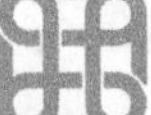

Servings : _______________

Ingredients:

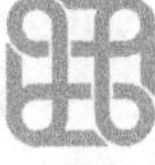
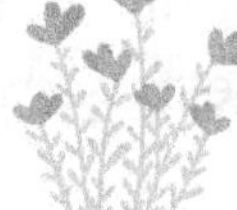

• 1 cup uncooked brown rice
• 2 tbsp olive oil
• 1 onion, sliced
• 2 cloves garlic, minced
• 1 red bell pepper, sliced
• 1 cup broccoli florets
• 1 cup sliced mushrooms
• 1 cup snow peas or snap peas
• 2 cups chopped kale or spinach
• 2 tbsp low•sodium soy sauce
• 1 tsp grated ginger
• 1/4 tsp red pepper flakes (optional)
• Salt and pepper to taste

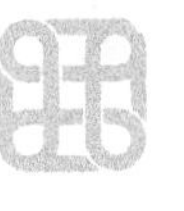
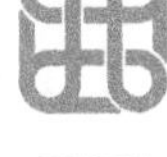
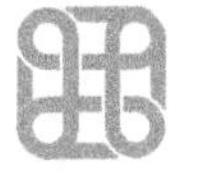

Is the recipe easy to follow?

113. *Vegetable Stir•Fry with Brown Rice*

1. Cook the brown rice according to package instructions.

2. In a large skillet or wok, heat the olive oil over medium•high heat. Add the onion and garlic and sauté for 2•3 minutes until fragrant.

3. Add the bell pepper, broccoli, mushrooms, and snow peas. Stir•fry for 5•7 minutes until vegetables are tender•crisp.

4. Stir in the kale/spinach, soy sauce, ginger, and red pepper flakes (if using). Cook for 2•3 minutes until greens are wilted.

5. Season with salt and pepper to taste.

6. Serve the vegetable stir•fry over the cooked brown rice.

This dish is packed with fiber, vitamins, and minerals, making it a great option for a diabetic•friendly, senior•friendly meal. The brown rice provides complex carbs and the vegetables are low in carbs and high in nutrients.

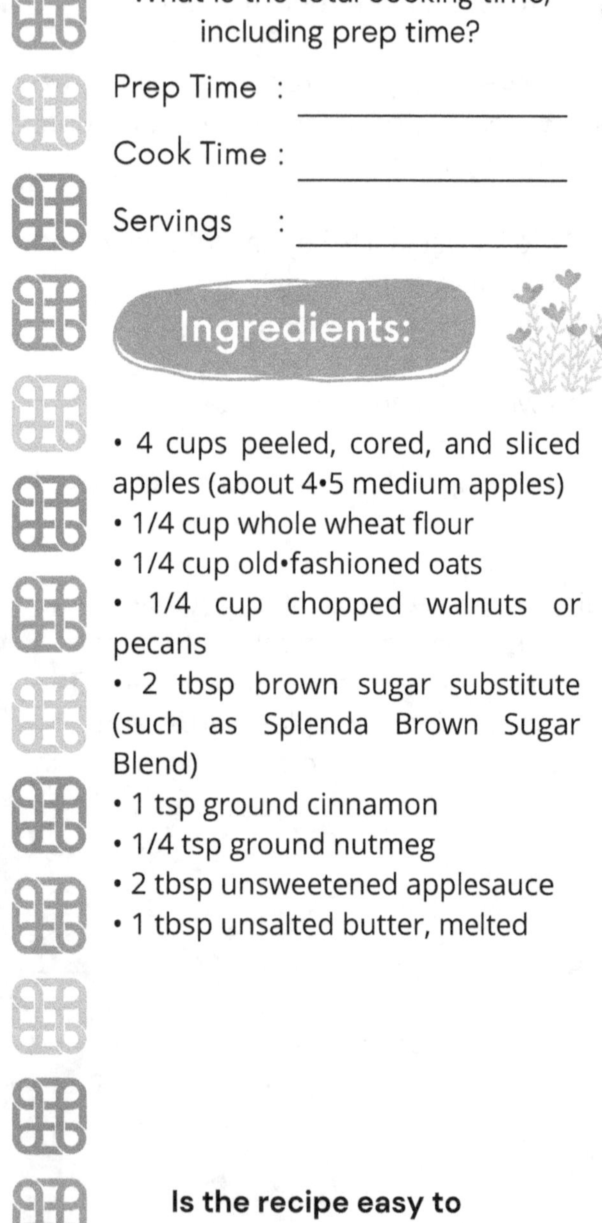

What is the total cooking time, including prep time?

Prep Time : _______________

Cook Time : _______________

Servings : _______________

Ingredients:

- 4 cups peeled, cored, and sliced apples (about 4•5 medium apples)
- 1/4 cup whole wheat flour
- 1/4 cup old•fashioned oats
- 1/4 cup chopped walnuts or pecans
- 2 tbsp brown sugar substitute (such as Splenda Brown Sugar Blend)
- 1 tsp ground cinnamon
- 1/4 tsp ground nutmeg
- 2 tbsp unsweetened applesauce
- 1 tbsp unsalted butter, melted

Is the recipe easy to follow?

114. Apple and Oatmeal Crisp

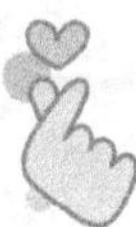

Procedure:

1. Preheat oven to 350°F. Lightly grease an 8x8 inch baking dish.

2. In a large bowl, toss the sliced apples with the whole wheat flour until the apples are evenly coated. Transfer to the prepared baking dish.

3. In a medium bowl, combine the oats, nuts, brown sugar substitute, cinnamon, and nutmeg. Stir in the applesauce and melted butter until the mixture is crumbly.

4. Sprinkle the oat topping evenly over the apples.

5. Bake for 30•35 minutes, until the apples are tender and the topping is golden brown.

6. Allow to cool for 10•15 minutes before serving.

This apple crisp is a healthier dessert option for diabetics and seniors. The whole wheat flour, oats, and nuts provide fiber, while the brown sugar substitute keeps the sugar content low. Apples and spices add natural sweetness without added sugars.

Serve warm, or chilled, and enjoy this comforting and nutritious treat!

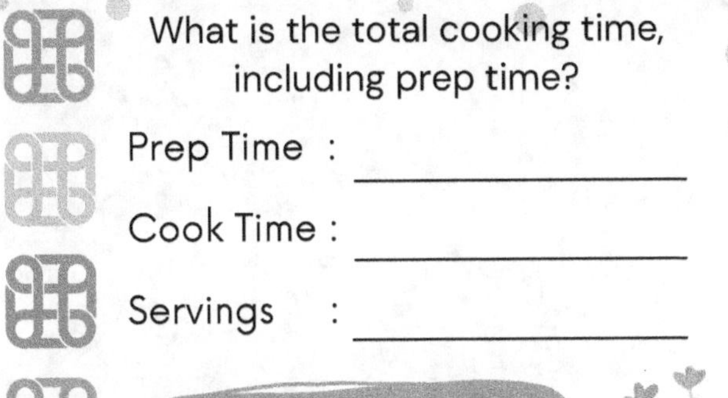

What is the total cooking time, including prep time?

Prep Time : _______________

Cook Time : _______________

Servings : _______________

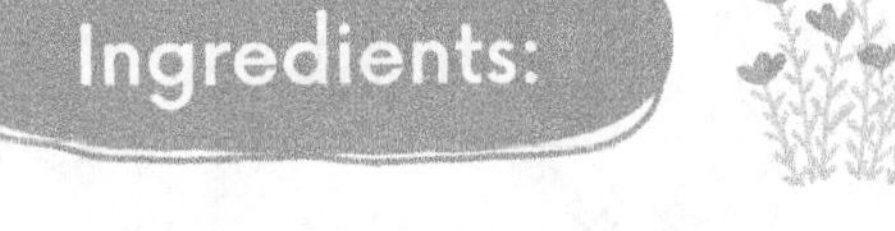

Ingredients:

- 1 (15 oz) can chickpeas (garbanzo beans), drained and rinsed
- 1 tbsp olive oil
- 1 tsp ground cumin
- 1 tsp paprika
- 1/2 tsp garlic powder
- 1/4 tsp salt
- 1/4 tsp black pepper

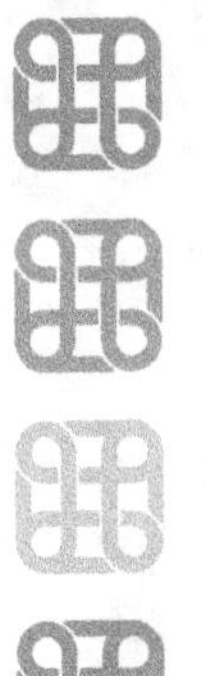

Is the recipe easy to follow?

115. Roasted Chickpeas

Procedure:

1. Preheat oven to 400°F. Line a baking sheet with parchment paper.

2. Pat the drained and rinsed chickpeas very dry with paper towels or a clean kitchen towel. This will help them get crispy.

3. In a medium bowl, toss the chickpeas with the olive oil, cumin, paprika, garlic powder, salt, and pepper until evenly coated.

4. Spread the chickpeas in a single layer on the prepared baking sheet.

5. Roast for 20•25 minutes, stirring halfway, until the chickpeas are crispy and golden brown.

6. Allow to cool for 5 minutes before serving.

Nutritional Benefits:
• Chickpeas are high in fiber, protein, and complex carbs, making them a great snack for diabetics.
• The spices add flavor without added sugars.
• Roasting the chickpeas makes them crispy and satisfying, similar to a crunchy snack.

This recipe is easy to make and a healthy alternative to traditional snacks. Roasted chickpeas make a great portable, high•protein snack for seniors with diabetes. Enjoy them on their own or use them as a topping for salads, soups, or other dishes.